BUILDING GOOD SPEECH

Word Lists for

[s, z, ʃ , ʒ , tʃ , dʒ , θ, ð, l, r, k, g, f, v]

Kathleen Pendergast

Supervisor, Speech and Hearing

Seattle Public Schools

731C1

STANWIX HOUSE, INC.

PITTSBURGH, PENNSYLVANIA

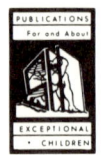

Published simultaneously in Canada by
J. M. Dent & Sons (Canada) Ltd.
Toronto, Ontario

First printing—November 1971
Second printing—August 1972

ISBN 0-87076-855-7
Library of Congress Catalog Card Number: 77-148146

Phonetic Alphabet Symbols
Used in
BUILDING GOOD SPEECH

Consonants

[s]	sue	[z]	zoo
[ʃ]	shook	[ʒ]	usual
[tʃ]	cheer	[dʒ]	jeer
[θ]	thank	[ð]	than
[l]	lip	[r]	rip
[k]	come	[g]	gum
[f]	fine	[v]	vine
[ŋ]	ring		

Vowels

[i]	key	[ʊ]	could
[ɪ]	kit	[u]	coo
[e]	cane	[ʌ]	cut
[ɛ]	kettle	[ə]	cadet
[æ]	cat	[ɝ]	anchor
[ɑ]	cot	[ɜ]*	cur
[ɔ]	caught	[ɝ]	cur
[o]	coat		

Diphthongs

[aɪ]	kite	[ɔɪ]	coy
[aʊ]	cow	[ju]	cue

*Eastern and Southern

INTRODUCTION

Speech clinicians are constantly seeking better methods of articulation therapy. BUILDING GOOD SPEECH suggests a slightly different approach to the correction of articulatory defects. It groups words according to their phonetic environment and suggests that if a client is able to say a certain sound combination easily, he should have little difficulty incorporating that combination into all the words which contain it if the words are presented in an orderly sequence. This book is based on the learning theory of progressing from the known to the unknown. That is, it provides the material to progress from the sound in isolation to a systematic presentation of the sound in all possible positions in a word.

Many speech clinicians teach a sound in isolation and then in nonsense syllables in combination with vowels. They frequently find that the sound combined with a particular vowel or another consonant is easiest for the client, but they do not always capitalize on this finding because they have not had adequate practice material organized in this manner.

Traditional speech therapy materials list words with a sound in the initial, medial, and final positions but cognizance of the phonetic environment of the sound is frequently lacking. The words *answer* (consonant + $[s]$ + vowel), *bobsled* (consonant + $[s]$ + consonant), *rooster* (vowel + $[s]$ + consonant), and *missing* (vowel + $[s]$ + vowel) are all medial $[s]$ words but represent different levels of difficulty for a client with a defective $[s]$.

In this book, the words are listed according to their phonetic environment* not only to provide readily accessible practice material, but also to identify areas of the client's strengths and weaknesses.

Because clients differ in their ability to produce a sound in various phonetic environments, it is recommended that the speech clinician test to find the easiest combination and begin there. For example, a small child who substitutes a $[t]$ for a $[s]$ frequently will have difficulty with words in the $[s]$ + Vowel section and will say *stee* for *see*, *staw* for *saw*, etc. However, he might have little or no difficulty with initial $[s]$ blends or with words in the Vowel + $[s]$ section. These words should be practiced until the sound is stabilized and usually when words from the $[s]$ + Vowel section are introduced later, little difficulty is encountered.

If a client who has a defective $[s]$ is able to say a $[s]$ which is preceded by a vowel more easily than a $[s]$ which is followed by a vowel,

*Phonetic environment refers to the phonemes which precede and follow the sound being taught. For example, the $[s]$ in *missing* and the $[s]$ in *kissing* have the same phonetic environment $[ɪsɪ]$ while the phonetic environment of *lipstick* $[pst]$ is different.

To Bill

CONTENTS

there are many words to practice in the Vowel + [s] section. Clients also find that the sound in combination with a particular vowel sound is easier than the sound in combination with other vowel sounds. For example, [is] may be easier than [us]. When this has been determined, adequate practice material may be found in this book because the words are listed according to vowels.

When the sound combination has been practiced until it is stabilized, a slight shift in the vowel sound usually creates no difficulty. If the client can say *niece, lease,* and *piece* easily, he should be able to say *hiss, kiss,* and *miss* but might have more trouble, initially, with *goose* and *moose.*

It was stated earlier that the approach to articulation therapy suggested in this book is proceeding from the known to the unknown. For this reason, not all words containing the sound in the medial position are listed together. They are listed according to the position of the vowel or other consonant in relation to the sound. If it is desirable to teach the word *uncertain,* to a client who has a defective [s] and has already learned *sir* and *certain,* a quick review of the latter two will usually bring success.

Because the words are listed according to vowels, they are particularly useful for clients with foreign accents. When a consonant sound is being taught, difficult vowels and diphthongs may be avoided at the beginning of therapy and introduced later when the sound has been mastered. Or the lists may be used for vowel or diphthong practice only.

There are three sections in the introduction to the lists of words for each sound.

1. Construction of the Word Lists

The categories for each sound are listed to aid the clinician in locating the type of words required. The categories often are as follow:

a. The sound followed by a vowel including the sound in the initial position and initial and medial blends.
b. The sound preceded by a vowel including the sound in the final position and final and medial blends.
c. The sound preceded and followed by a vowel.
d. Final and medial blends.

The sound is usually combined with vowels and diphthongs in the order which follows:

[i, ɪ, e, ɛ, aɪ, æ, ɑ, ɔ, o, ʊ, u, ʌ, ə, ɝ, ɜ, ɚ, aʊ, ɔɪ, ju]

Where appropriate, the sound is usually combined with other consonants in the order which follows:

[h, j, r, k, g, ŋ, t, d, n, l, s, z, ʃ, ʒ, tʃ, dʒ, p, b, m, f, v, θ, ð, hw, w]

For example, this is illustrated through the words sake, sane, sale, sage, same, safe, save; or race, case, lace, chase, pace, base, face, vase. An understanding of the order of listing is important for best use of the book. If words with a slight shift in the vowel sounds are wanted, such words as seek, sick, sake, sack, sock, and suck are found near the beginning of the [s] + Vowel lists because [s] is combined with [k] after [h, j, r].

The words are incorporated into the lists in a specific manner. Except for [h, j, r], the sounds which are combined with the sound being studied are articulated in the back of the mouth first and then move forward to the front of the mouth and the lips. If the clinician needs practice material to stabilize the [saɪ], words such as *sight, side,* and *sign,* which require the same tongue movement, might be easier initially than *siren, cider,* and *syphon* and they are easily found in the lists. Also, if the client has other defective sounds, the clinician may wish to avoid words containing both the sound being studied and another defective sound. For example, if the sound being studied is [s] and the client also has a defective [r], the clinician might want to avoid words at the beginning of the [s] lists because [r] is combined with [s] after [h, j].

In most of the lists, if the sound appears twice in a word, the second sound is underlined.

In the lists, most words ending with s, ed, er, ly, and ing are not listed but if additional words are needed in the Sound + Vowel section, these endings should be considered. In the Vowel + Sound section, words ending with s and ed are not listed but should be used for final blend practice. In the Vowel + Sound + Vowel section, if additional words are needed for [ɪ], add ing, and sometimes es, to the appropriate words in the Vowel + Sound section.

2. Characteristics and Use of the Word Lists

The words in this book are not limited to children's vocabulary and, therefore, are not appropriate for all clients. They are listed to allow the clinician more flexibility when working with adults and also to show the relative frequency of each sound combination. There are many more words beginning with [sʌ] than with [sɔɪ], for example.

Obviously, not all words containing a sound are listed, but those used provide a representative sample.

The listing of the words is based on standard American speech, according to Kenyon and Knott[*] or Carrell and Tiffany,[†] and, therefore, not all lists will be appropriate in all geographic sections where local dialects may influence pronunciation.

While many clinicians teach a sound in the traditional initial, final, and medial positions, there are many children with inconsistent misarticulations who can already say the sound in a particular phonetic environment. It is wise for the speech clinician to test the various phonetic environments and if the phonetic environment where the sound is said correctly can be identified, begin therapy there. The location of the word lists for the initiation of therapy for each phonetic environment is noted in each section.

Depending upon the age and ability of the client, it may or may not be advisable to proceed down the lists of Sound + Vowel or Vowel + Sound through the medial blends. If not, skip to the next list.

3. Methods of Correcting the Sound

There are many excellent books which give detailed descriptions of how sounds are produced. Therefore, this information is not repeated here but some of the important aspects which should be noted if the sound is taught by a placement method are included.

It is suggested in each section that the sound be taught by the auditory-visual method. This method is based on ear training and sound discrimination which are not included in this book. When the client is proficient in the auditory aspect of a sound, the clinician says the sound and asks the client to repeat it. This is the natural way a sound is learned and should always be attempted first. It should be noted here that the importance of a perfect model is paramount. When attempting to show the client the position of the tongue for some sounds, the clinician must open his mouth fairly wide. Most sounds made in this position are faulty and should not be used as models for the client to imitate. If the client is unable to produce a sound, the fault may lie in the model presented by the speech clinician rather than in the client.

It is often inadvisable in the initial stages of therapy to present

---

[*]J.S. Kenyon and T.A. Knott, *A Pronouncing Dictionary of American English* (Springfield, Mass., G. & C. Merriam Co., 1949).

[†]J. Carrell and W.R. Tiffany, *Phonetics: Theory and Application to Speech Improvement* (New York, McGraw-Hill, Inc., 1960).

words which contain both the defective sound and the sound formerly substituted for it. An example of this is the word south or this for a protrusional lisper, cat or tack for a client whose substitution is [t/k], and god or dog for a client whose substitution is [d/g]. Naturally, these words will be presented later when the sound is stabilized, but they might cause needless frustration if they are presented too soon.

If the articulation of professional speakers, such as television news announcers, is observed carefully, it will be noted that their teeth are clearly visible most of the time. Conversely, speakers with careless articulation frequently cover their teeth with their lips. Often the clinician will teach the exact position of the tongue for the production of a sound and yet a fuzzy sound emerges. Many times it is the result of of the lips, particularly the lower lip, interfering with the breath stream. This is especially true with the sibilant sounds [s, z, ʃ, ʒ, tʃ, dʒ]. The lips are so important in articulation therapy that the speech clinician should be cognizant of their position at all times.

It is the earnest desire of the author that the word lists in BUILDING GOOD SPEECH will aid many speech clinicians in planning lessons which build on the client's strengths so gradually that frustration is never experienced in the therapy sessions.

[s]

Construction of the [s] *Word Lists*

1. There are six categories:
    a. the [s] followed by a vowel including initial [s] and medial [s] blends.
    b. initial, medial, and final [s] blends [s m, s p, s p r, s p l, s t, s t r, s n, s l, s k, s k r, s k w, s w, sh, s ʃ, s t ʃ, sf, s hw].
    c. final [s] blends [t s, n t s, l t s, r t s, p s, m p s, r s, f s, k s, ŋ k s].
    d. the [s] preceded by a vowel including final [s] and final and medial [s] blends.
    e. the [s] preceded and followed by a vowel.
    f. some [s] words which might be difficult at the beginning of therapy.

2. Where appropriate, the [s] is combined with other consonants in the order which follows:
    [h, j, r, k, g, ŋ, t, d, n, l, ʃ, ʒ, tʃ, dʒ, p, b, m, f, v, hw, w].
    The words sake, sane, sale, sage, same, safe, save; or race, case, lace, chase, pace, face, and vase illustrate some of the combinations. If a slight shift in vowels is desired, words such as seek, sick, sake, sack, sock, soak, and suck are found near the beginning of the lists because [s] is combined with [k] after [h, j, r].

3. Where appropriate, the [s] is combined with vowels and diphthongs in the order which follows:
    [i, ɪ, e, ɛ, aɪ, æ, ɑ, ɔ, o, ʊ, u, ʌ, ə, ɚ, ɝ, ʒ, aʊ, ɔɪ, ju].

4. To facilitate the location of words in a category, medial [s] words are noted by xx.

Characteristics and Use of the [s] *Word Lists*

1. Choose words which are appropriate for the age and interests of the client. Many words are listed for high school students and adults but would not be considered for small children. The lists also reflect the relative frequency of each vowel in combination with [s]. For example, there are many more words beginning with [s ʌ] than [s ɔɪ].

2. Determine which sound combination is the easiest.
    a. If it is the [s] + Vowel, begin on pages 6—9. Choose the vowel which makes [s] production easiest.

1

b. If it is initial [s] blends, begin on pages 10–13. Choose the blend which is the easiest. Frequently this is [s m] or [s p].

c. If it is Vowel + [s], begin on pages 19–23. Choose the vowel which makes [s] production easiest.

d. If it is a final [s] blend, begin on pages 14–18. Often the [t s, n t s] or the [p s, m p s] blends are easiest.

3. It may or may not be desirable to proceed down the [s] + Vowel lists through the medial blends. If it is not, skip to the next list. If they are presented later and prove to be difficult, a quick review of the initial [s] words should make the medial [s] blends easier. For example, if *uncertain* is presented, a quick review of *sir* and *certain* should prove to be all that is necessary for correct production of *uncertain*. This also is true of the medial [s] words in the Vowel + [s] section.

Methods of Correcting the [s] Sound

The tongue blade and the alveolar ridge are used to produce the [s] sound. The aperture for the air stream is made with the tongue blade at the central apex of the alveolar ridge and hard palate. The portion of the tongue blade used is partly dependent upon the antero-postero width of the alveolar ridge and partly dependent upon the position of the tongue tip. The tongue tip may be elevated to a position behind, but not touching, the upper central incisors, it may be behind the lower central incisors, or it may be at a point between these two positions. Position of the tongue tip during production of [s] may be checked by inserting a wooden coffee stirrer or one-fourth inch wooden peg vertically between the upper and lower molars. The [s] sound produced in this manner will not be clear but production can be observed.

One of the most important aspects of producing a sharp [s] sound is the position of the lower lip. It must be pulled down and the lower teeth must be clearly visible or the [s] will be fuzzy.

The auditory visual method of teaching the [s] is preferred and should be attempted first. However, some clients are unable to say the [s] without additional assistance. The following suggested ideas have been helpful in these instances.

If a placement method is used, the elevated tongue tip production of [s] usually should be attempted first because [s] and [z] frequently are combined with other tongue tip sounds [t, d, n, l] in words and conversation, and less tongue adjustment is required if the [s] also is produced with the tongue tip elevated. However, some clients find it easier to place the tongue tip behind the lower central incisors, particularly if

2

they have a very wide alveolar ridge. If an acoustically acceptable [s] is produced, it is unimportant whether the tongue tip is up or down.

1. Ask the client to close his teeth, as if he were chewing, and blow. Check the closure to be sure the molars are occluded. When using this method, it usually is not necessary to call attention to the tongue position if a good [s] sound results. Use a mirror if any difficulty is encountered.

2. If the client has difficulty saying a clear sound, often the suggestion to "smile hard" produces the desired results. Apparently the tensing of the mouth muscles encourages tensing of the tongue muscles which results in a clear[s].

3. A Method of Correcting a Lateral or Protrusional Lisp

   a. Ask the client to say [t] very quietly, but sharply, and with as little tongue movement as possible. Only the very tip of the tongue should move. There should be no vowel sound after the [t] to keep the tongue in the correct position. (The two errors which many beginning speech clinicians make when using this method are both in the area of providing a perfect model. Either their [t] is quiet but not sharp and is really not a good [t] sound or they add a vowel [tʌ] which brings the tongue tip away from the alveolar ridge and makes the method useless.)
   b. Ask the client to say [t] quietly and let a little breath come after it[ts]. Demonstrate. Do not tell a person with a lateral lisp that he will say [s] or he will revert to his distortion. At first the [s] may be very faint and fuzzy. Strengthen it by making a sharper [t]. The suggestion "hit the [t] harder" may be helpful. Practice the[ts]. Be sure the lower lip does not cover the lower central incisors or the [s] will not be clear. At this point, check the air stream to be sure that it is emitted centrally. This may be done by holding a drinking straw against the cutting edge of the upper central incisors. Move the straw along the cutting edge of the upper teeth until the point of emission is located.
   c. Ask the client to prolong the [ɪ] sound and then add[ts]. Gradually shorten the [ɪ] until the client says *it's*. If the client reverts to a lateral or protrusional[s], go back to the [ts] and tell him this is the sound to add to the [ɪ]. Put the word in short sentences which do not contain other [s]words such as these: It's raining. It's pretty. It's cold. It's hot.

3

d. Practice the final [ts] blends on page 14. Use the words in sentences which do not have other [s] words.

e. Ask the client to say [ts], pause, and without changing the position of the tongue say [s]. Practice [ts−s].

f. Ask the client to say [s]. Sometimes the suggestion to "think" [t] but only say the [s] is helpful. If at any point the client reverts to the lateral or protrusional [s], go back to the [ts] and gradually build until a clear [s] can be produced.

g. At this point, some people find Vowel + [s] words easier. If so, practice the words on pages 19−23. Others find initial [s] blends easier. If so, practice the words on pages 10−13. Still others find [s] + Vowel words easier. If so, practice the words on pages 6−9.

h. The Vowel + [s] + Vowel words on pages 24−25 are usually the most difficult and probably would be practiced last.

4. Use the method described in number 3 above but substitute the following:

a. [nt]

b. [nts]

c. Ask the client to prolong [hɪ] then add [nts]. Gradually shorten the vowel until he says *hints*.

d. Practice the final [nts] blends on pages 14−15. Then practice the final [ts] blends on page 14. The suggestion to "think" [n] but only say [ts] may be helpful if the client retains the [n] on the [ts] words.

e. Proceed with steps e to h above.

5. For a client who substitutes [t] for [s], the [s] blends, particularly [sm] and [sp], on page 10 are usually the easiest. However, Vowel + [s] words on pages 19−23 may be easier for some clients. Either of these groups of words tends to inhibit the addition of the [t] after the [s] which very young children frequently add in [s] + Vowel words as in *stun* for *sun* or *stee* for *see*.

6. Ask the client to repeat the [t] sound, with no vowel added, several times very rapidly. It is impossible to do this without saying [s] between each [t] if the [t] is said correctly. Draw the attention of the client to the sharp [s] sound. Isolate it.

4

7.   Ask the client to "whistle" with a series of [p s] sounds. Ask him to say one [p s]. Practice the final [p s] blends on pages 15—16.

8.   Ask the client to prolong the [θ] sound as he gradually pulls his tongue in and slides his tongue tip up the posterior surface of the upper central incisors to the alveolar ridge. Often the [s] sound is the result.

9.   Ask the client to prolong the [i] sound and gradually raise his tongue tip. The resulting sound often will be [z]. Ask him to whisper the [z] to produce [s].

10.   Place about one inch of an applicator on the central groove of the client's tongue. Ask him to close his teeth, raise his tongue tip to the alveolar ridge, and blow. Use the pressure necessary to maintain the central groove. Gradually pull the applicator forward and out to determine whether or not he can maintain the central groove. Ask the client to place the applicator on his tongue and repeat the actions above.

11.   When using any of the above methods, it is very important to have the client maintain his natural bite when producing the [s] if this is at all possible. If he must swing his jaw in or out to say [s], it is questionable whether or not he will retain the new sound after leaving therapy. Partly for cosmetic reasons, it is particularly important not to swing the jaw to one side or the other. In clients with severe overjets, it may be necessary not only to push the jaw forward but also to use the lower lip to produce a sound which approximates the [s]. However, these cases are rare and require the exception rather than the rule for correction.

[s] + Vowel*

[si]

sea	cereal	similar	seine
see	serial	symptom	saint
seek	syringe	simple	sale
secret	sick	symbol	sail
sequin	secure	symphony	sailer
sequence	seclude	sift	sailor
sequel	cigar	sieve	sailcloth
seat	cigarette	civic	sage
seed	signal	civil	saber
cedar	signature		sable
seen	signify	**xx**	same
scene	sing		safe
senior	sink	taxi	safekeeping
senile	single	galaxy	safeguard
seal	singular	pixy	safety
ceiling	sit	insecure	safety pin
seashore	city	insignia	save
siege	citron	incision	savor
seep	sedate	insipid	savory
seam	sin	pensive	
seem	synonym	rancid	**xx**
seaman	cinema	transit	
seaweed	cinnamon	dancing	unsafe
	cinder	fancy	compensate
xx	cinch	uncivil	fiancé
	singe	currency	wholesale
exceed	sill	consider	lifesaver
cottonseed	silly	gypsy	
unseeing	cylinder	homesick	### [sɛ]
unseat	syllable		
unseen	silk	### [se]	ceremony
unseal	silt		cerebral
	silver	say	serape
### [sɪ]	situate	sake	second
	sip	sacred	secular
sierra		sane	secretary
sear			

---

*Most words ending with er, ed, ing, and ly are not included and should be considered if additional words are desired.

sect
section
segregate
segment
set
setter
settle
said
sediment
senate
sent
cent
center
sentinel
centipede
sentiment
centimeter
central
sentry
send
century
sell
cell
cellar
celery
celluloid
celebrate
cellophane
celt
seldom
self
selfish
selvage
session
separate
September
cemetery
seminary
seminar

sever
several
seven
seventeen

xx

ourself
yourself
excel
except
accent
accelerate
acceleration
accept
itself
insect
inset
onset
unsettle
unselfish
consent
upset
absent
himself

[saɪ]

sigh
sire
siren
cycle
cyclone
sight
site
cite
citation
side
cider
sign

silo
silent
silage
cipher
siphon
syphon

xx

foresight
excite
excitable
oxide
outside
broadside
hindsight
insight
inside
unsightly
unsigned
hillside

[sæ]

sac
sack
saccharin
sackful
sag
sang
sank
sanction
sanctuary
sat
satire
Saturday
sateen
satin
satinwood
satellite
sad

sadden
saddle
sanity
sanitary
sanatorium
sand
sandal
sandpaper
sandbag
sandman
sandwich
Sally
sallow
salary
salad
salamander
salutation
salvia
salvage
sash
sashay
sachet
saturate
satchel
sap
sapling
sabotage
salmon
sample
sampler
sapphire
salve
savvy
savage

xx

insanity
unsaddle
unsanitary

7

[sɑ]

sahib
sari
sorrow
sardine
sergeant
sock
soccer
socket
soggy
saga
sod
solder
sodden
sonnet
solitaire
solitary
solid
soluble
solemn
solve
sob
somber
sombrero
sophomore
sovereign

xx

corsage
insomnia
absolve

[sɔ]

saw
sorry
sorrel
sorghum
sort
sordid

song
sought
saunter
salt
soft
soften

xx

bucksaw
jigsaw
unsalted
absorb

[so]

so
sow
sew
soar
sore
soak
soke
soda
sodium
sole
soul
solo
solar
sold
soldier
social
socialite
sociable
sojourn
soap
sober
sofa
soviet

xx

torso
insole
insolate
console
unsold
unsociable
also

[su]

sue
Sue
suet
suit
suitor
suitable
soon
suture
soup
super
superb
superman
soufflé
souvenir
sewer

xx

unsuited
unsuitable
consume
chop suey

[sʌ]

suck
sucker
succotash
suckling
suction

sung
sunk
subtle
sudden
son
sun
sonny
sunup
sundae
Sunday
sundown
sundry
sunlight
sunshine
sunburn
sunfish
sunflower
sully
sullen
sulk
sultan
sultry
sulfate
such
sup
supper
supple
supplement
sub
suburb
sublet
sublimate
subject
submarine
subway
sum
some
summer

8

summary
summertime
summit
summon
somehow
sometime
somebody
somewhere
somewhat
someway
someone
suffer
suffocate

xx

midsummer
insult
unsung
grandson
consult

[sə]

sorority
sarong
serene
surrender
surround
ceramic
succumb
sagacious
sonata
select
salute
solidity
solidify
solution

celebrity
saliva
superior
superlative
support
subpoena
soprano
supreme
supply
sublime
subject
submerge
submit
cement
semantic
safari
severe
severity
civilian

xx

varsity
accident
hexagon
oxygen
flexible
approximate
catsup
incident
insulate
insulation
consolation
insulin
principle
principal
lonesome

ransom
handsome
intensify
wholesome
balsam
meddlesome
rhapsody
absolute

[sɚ]

certificate
surmount
survey
surveyor
survive
survival

xx

answer
cancer
dancer
ulcer

[sɝ]

sir
syrup
cirque
circuit
circular
circulate
circulation
circle
certain
certitude
certify
certification

surname
surly
sirloin
search
surcharge
serge
surge
surgical
surgeon
sermon
serf
surf
serve
survey
servant

xx

insert
insertion
uncertain
conserve

[sau]

sow
sour
sauerkraut
sound

xx

unsound

[sɔɪ]

soy
soil

xx

unsoiled

Initial, Medial, and Final [s] Blends

[sm]

smear
smitten
smell
smelt
smite
smile
smack
smatter
smash
smashup
smart
smock
small
smoke
smote
smolder
smug
smuggle
smudge
smirk
smirch

[sp]

speak
speed
speech
spear
spirit
spin
spinach
spill
spade
Spain
spare
speck
speckle
sped
spent

spend
spell
special
spy
spire
spite
spike
spider
spine
sparrow
spank
spangle
spatter
span
spark
sparkle
spot
spoke
sport
spoon
spool
spunk
spun
spaghetti
spurt
spoil

xx

experiment
expect
expel
expand
expert
export
larkspur
outspoken
inspect

transport
unspoken
unspoiled
conspire
tablespoon

[spr]

spree
sprig
spring
sprinkle
sprint
spray
sprain
spread
spry
sprang
sprawl
sprung
sprout

xx

bedspread

[spl]

spleen
split
splint
splinter
splender
splendid
splatter
splash
splotch
splurge

xx

horseplay
explore

[st]

steer
steal
steep
steam
stick
sting
still
stilt
stitch
stiff
stay
steak
state
stadium
stain
stale
station
stage
stable
stair
stead
steady
step
stem
sty
style
stack
stag
stand
statue
stab
stamp
staff

10

star	taxed	strip	sniffle
stark	waxed	stray	snake
start	boxed	straight	snail
starch	midst	strain	snare
starve	against	strange	snack
stock		stranger	snag
stocking	horsetail	stretch	snatch
stop	exterior	strike	snap
stork	external	stride	snarl
storm	trickster	stripe	snob
stalk	extent	strap	snow
stall	extend	straw	snore
store	backstage	strong	snoot
story	bedstead	strawberry	snoop
stone	instant	stroke	snug
stole	instead	stroll	snub
stove	unsteady	struck	snuff
stood	unstable	struggle	
stew	monster	strung	xx
stool	cornstarch		
stuck	bolster	xx	arson
stung	candlestick		vixen
study	chopstick	extreme	oxen
stun	lipstick	extra	
stunt	lobster	extract	parsnip
stomach	abstain	backstroke	vaccinate
stump	hamster	construct	unsnarl
stuff	homestead	construction	unsnap
stir	hemstitch	constrict	
stern	drumstick	demonstrate	[sl]
stout	beefsteak	obstruct	
		abstract	sleek
xx	[str]		sleet
		[sn]	sleep
mixed	streak		sleeve
fixed	street	sneer	slick
text	stream	sneak	sling
context	string	snip	slink
next	strict	sniff	slit
			slip

slim
sliver
sleigh
slate
slain
slave
sled
sledge
slept
sly
slight
slide
slack
slang
slat
slant
slash
slap
slab
slam
slot
slop
slaw
slow
slope
slug
slush
slum
slump
slumber
slouch

xx

parcel
morsel
tinsel
pencil

cancel
consul
capsule

parsley
porcelain
horselaugh
backslide
translate
counselor
bobsled

[sk]

ski
skier
scheme
skit
skid
skin
skill
skip
skim
skimp
skate
skein
scale
scare
scary
skeleton
sketch
sky
scat
scatter
scan
scant
scandal
scalp
scab
scamp

scar
scarlet
scarf
Scotch
scald
scoff
score
scone
scold
scope
scoot
school
scoop
skunk
skull

xx

excursion
buckskin
unskilled
hopscotch
obscure
exclude
exclaim

[skr]

screen
screech
scream
script
scribble
scrimp
scrape
scratch
scrap
scram
scramble

scrawl
scroll
screw
Scrooge
scrub

xx

unscramble
unscrew

[skw]

squeak
squeal
squint
square
squat
squad
squander
squash
squab
squabble
squaw
squawk
squall
squirt
squirrel
squirm

[sw]

sweet
suite
Swede
sweep
swing
swish
switch
swim

[s h]

swift	swab	xx	mixture
sway	swamp		texture
suede	suave	exhale	
swear	swarm	falsehood	[s f]
sweat	swore		
swell	swollen	[s ʃ]	xx
swelter	swung		
swipe	swum	xx	horsefly
swag	swirl		henceforth
swang	swerve	horseshoe	transfer
swam			
swat		[s tʃ]	[s hw]
swan	xx		
swallow		xx	xx
swap	unswerving	exchange	horsewhip
			elsewhere

Final [s] Blends

[t s]

[i]

		[ɑ]	
eats	mates	rots	ruts
heats	waits	trots	cuts
greets		cots	nuts
treats	[ɛ]	tots	shuts
cleats	frets	dots	putts
pleats	gets	knots	mutts
sheets	nets	lots	
cheats	lets	plots	[ɝ]
repeats	jets	blots	
beats	pets	shots	hurts
meats	bets	jots	dirts
defeats	vets	pots	blurts
wheats	wets	watts	flirts
			shirts

[ɪ]

	[aɪ]	[o]	[n t s]
its	heights	oats	[ɪ]
hits	rights	coats	
grits	fright	goats	hints
kits	kites	totes	rinse
tickets	tights	notes	prints
knits	nights	gloats	prince
pits	lights	bloats	tints
bits	flights	floats	chintz
rabbits	bites	boats	mints
mitts	fights	moats	mince
fits		votes	wince

[e]

	[æ]	[u]	[e]
hates	hats	hoots	paints
rates	rats	roots	faints
crates	cats	fruits	
grates	tats	toots	[ɛ]
traits	gnats	loots	
gates	flats	flutes	hence
dates	chats	shoots	rents
plates	pats	boots	tense
baits	bats		tents
	mats	[ʌ]	
	vats	huts	

14

pretense
intense
dents
dense
pence
commence
fence
offense
defense
whence

[æ]

rants
prance
France
dance
finance
lance
glance
chance
pants
romance
advance

[ɑ]

wants

[ʌ]

hunts
dunce
punts
bunts
once

[ə]

recurrence
ignorance

conference
entrance
elegance
independence
ambulance
allowance
frequence

[aʊ]

ounce
trounce
announce
pronounce
flounce
pounce
bounce

[l t s]
[ɪ]

kilts
guilts
tilts
wilts
quilts

[ɛ]

else
pelts
belts
melts
welts

[ɔ]

halts
malts

faults
false
waltz

[o]

colts
bolts
volts

[ʌ]

pulse
repulse

[r t s]
[ɑ]

arts
hearts
carts
tarts
darts
charts
parts
marts

[ɔ]

shorts
warts

[o]

courts
ports
airports
forts

[p s]
[i]

heaps
reaps

creeps
keeps
leaps
jeeps
peeps
beeps
weeps

[ɪ]

hips
rips
trips
drips
tips
dips
nips
lips
clips
eclipse
flips
ships
chips
whips

[e]

apes
grapes
drapes
capes
gapes
shapes

[aɪ]

gripes
types
pipes
wipes

15

[æ]

perhaps
raps
traps
caps
gaps
taps
naps
lapse
relapse
collapse
claps
flaps
chaps
maps

[ɑ]

hops
crops
drops
props
cops
tops
plops
flops
shops
chops
pops
mops

[o]

hopes
ropes
gropes
copes
dopes
lopes

16

popes
mopes

[u]

hoops
groups
troops
droops
coops
dupes
loops

[ʌ]

cups
pups

[mps]
[ɪ]

imps
crimps
shrimps
primps
limps
glimpse
blimps

[æ]

amps
ramps
cramps
tramps
tamps
lamps
clamps

champs
vamps

[ʌ]

humps
trumps
dumps
lumps
clumps
chumps
jumps
pumps
bumps
mumps

[rs]
[ɪ]

pierce
fierce

[ɔ]

horse
indorse
Norse

[o]

hoarse
coarse
course
recourse
force
enforce

[fs]
[i]

reefs
briefs
leafs
beliefs
chiefs
beefs

[ɪ]

ifs
tiffs
cliffs
biffs
miffs
whiffs

[e]

chafes
waifs

[ɛ]

chefs

[aɪ]

knife's
life's
wife's

[æ]

giraffes
graphs
laughs
chaffs

[ɔ]

cough
troughs

[u]

hoofs
roofs
proofs
goofs

[ʌ]

huffs
cuffs
bluffs
fluffs
puffs
buffs
muffs

[ks]
[i]

reeks
creeks
leaks
sheiks
cheeks
peaks
beaks
weeks

[ɪ]

hicks
kicks
ticks
Dick's
appendix
nix
nicks
licks
clicks
flicks

chicks
picks
mix
fix
prefix

[e]

aches
rakes
breaks
brakes
cakes
takes
lakes
flakes
shakes
bakes
makes
fakes
wakes

[ɛ]

hex
wrecks
treks
decks
index
necks
annex
triplex
duplex
complex
flecks
flex
checks
pecks
vex

[aɪ]

hikes
trikes
dikes
likes
bikes
mikes

[æ]

ax
pickax
racks
cracks
tracks
tacks
tax
lax
relax
flax
shacks
jacks
packs
backs
climax
wax

[ɑ]

ox
rocks
crocks
cocks
docks
knocks
locks
clocks
phlox
shocks

pox
box
fox

[ɔ]

talks
chalks
walks

[o]

hoax
croaks
coax
cloaks
chokes
jokes
pokes
folks

[ʊ]

hooks
crooks
brooks
cooks
nooks
looks
books

[ʌ]

trucks
tux
ducks
lux
clucks

17

[iŋ]

plucks	inks	kinks	jinx
shucks	rinks	lynx	minx
pucks	drinks	clinks	winks
	shrinks	blinks	

Vowel + [s] *

[is]

crease	actress	crevice	bristle
increase	kiss	novice	epistle
grease	gratis		missile
geese	lattice	**xx**	whistle
niece	lettuce		crisp
lease	notice		lisp
release	practice	risk	wisp
police	apprentice	brisk	
valise	jaundice	frisk	
fleece	holiness	disc	mishap
peace	happiness	disk	glycerin
piece	finis	obelisk	frisky
obese	tennis	whisk	discard
	menace	wrist	discord
xx	wilderness	jurist	discover
	harness	forest	discount
east	furnace	interest	biscuit
yeast	likeness	biggest	whisker
priest	witness	dentist	prescription
least	goodness	eldest	description
beast	kindness	earnest	describe
feast	roundness	colonist	discrete
	Alice	columnist	discriminate
Easter	palace	list	hysteria
eastern	malice	blacklist	history
recent	careless	enlist	orchestra
decent	necklace	tempest	restore
teaspoon	bliss	mist	restrain
policeman	miss	chemist	interesting
policemen	amiss	fist	distant
	remiss	harvest	district
[ɪs]	promise	twist	destruction
	pumice	pistol	canister
hiss	aphis	christen	banister
licorice	office	listen	minister
tigress	preface	glisten	blister
mattress			

*Most words ending with ed are omitted and should be considered for [st] blends.

ballistic	apace	impress	pesky
register	base	guess	estimate
majesty	abase	less	yesterday
bestow	face	unless	restaurant
mister	efface	bless	crestfallen
mystery	boldface	chess	presto
mistake	vase	mess	testify
mystify		confess	destine
whistler	xx		destroy
whistling	haste	xx	majesty
wistful	taste		pester
Christian	paste	desk	domestic
mischief	waste	rest	fester
respect	hasten	arrest	festival
respond	basin	crest	investigate
crispy	mason	guest	investment
despair	hasty	test	western
despite	haystack	detest	fluorescent
whisper	tasty	contest	chestnut
misbehave	pasty	nest	messenger
	pastry	lest	desolate
[e s]	waster	chest	gesture
ace	wastepaper	jest	question
race	bracelet	digest	desperate
erase	baseball	pest	chessboard
grace	baseboard	best	guesswork
trace	casement	vest	
brace	basement	invest	
embrace		west	[aɪs]
case	[ɛs]	lesson	
pillowcase		wrestle	ice
bookcase	yes	trestle	rice
encase	regress	nestle	price
lace	progress	vessel	dice
place	dress		nice
fireplace	address	escort	lice
chase	press	Eskimo	mice
pace	repress	rescue	vice
	depress		

20

vise	ask	mascara	colossal
device	cask	masquerade	jostle
advice	task	mascot	apostle
twice	flask	masculine	fossil
	bask	aster	wasp
	mask	drastic	
xx	rascal	caster	hostile
	contrast	castoff	hostility
bison	cast	gastric	hostage
	caste	ghastly	roster
ice cream	overcast	catastrophe	costume
eyestrain	outcast	fantastic	nostril
bystander	last	nasty	apostrophe
isolate	blast	plaster	imposter
isolation	past	plastic	posture
icebox	mast	elastic	hospital
iceberg	fast	pastor	hospitable
iceboat	vast	master	prosper
iceman	fasten	bandmaster	prospect
	wrestle	mastic	
[æs]	castle	faster	[ɔs]
	tassel	passenger	
harass	asp	fascinate	cross
grass	hasp	gaslight	across
bluegrass	grasp	gasoline	toss
brass	gasp	vaseline	loss
gas	clasp	pasture	gloss
lass		aspirin	floss
alas	grasshopper	aspect	boss
class	classroom	passport	emboss
glass	fiasco	classmate	moss
hourglass	cascade	asphalt	
pass	casket	glassful	**xx**
impasse	gasket	glassware	
bass	Alaska		frost
mass	basket	[ɑs]	cost
amass	basketball	**xx**	holocaust
	basketful	docile	lost

21

[us]

austerity	use	brusque	combustible
ostrich	abuse	tusk	muster
frosty	profuse	dusk	mustang
frostbite	truce	musk	mustard
costly	goose	rust	mustn't
Boston	mongoose	crust	rustler
foster	deuce	trust	
crosspatch	introduce	gust	

[os]

curious

	produce	dust	hilarious
	deduce	just	glorious
[os]	noose	adjust	hideous
	loose	bust	alias
gross	juice	combust	nucleus
engross	papoose	must	devious
glucose	caboose	hustle	obvious
dose	moose	rustle	pious
diagnose		tussle	bias
close		bustle	genius
	xx	muscle	bilious
	roost	mussel	chorus
xx	loosen	husky	generous
		musket	dangerous
host	rooster	muscular	embarrass
roast	acoustic	muskmelon	humorous
coast	useful	rusty	glamorous
ghost		trusty	virus
toast	[ʌs]	frustrate	walrus
post		custard	caucus
outpost	us	custody	hocus
boast	plus	custom	crocus
most	pus	customer	locus
almost	bus	gusto	focus
	omnibus	industrial	carcass
grocery	muss	luster	bogus
poster	fuss	cluster	fungus
postpone		bluster	tortoise
postmark	xx	fluster	cactus
postman		justify	
bowstring	husk		
	rusk		

22

lotus	August	interstate	house
impetus	ballast	perspire	playhouse
heinous	breakfast	persuade	greenhouse
monotonous	comparison		grouse
bonus	moccasin		douse
minus	medicine	[ɝs]	louse
luminous	magnificent		blouse
callus		coerce	mouse
callous	escape	hearse	
zealous	telescope	curse	
jealous	mosquito	nurse	xx
atlas	esteem	purse	
precious	estate	reimburse	household
capricious	establish	commerce	mousehole
gracious	astonish	verse	housetop
vivacious	astute	reverse	roustabout
luscious	astern	perverse	houseboat
delicious	astound	inverse	houseful
officious	astray	converse	housework
vicious	astronomer		
anxious	photostat		[ɔɪs]
outrageous	devastate	xx	
octopus	industry		choice
compass	illustrate		rejoice
pompous	illustration	burst	voice
Columbus	asleep	first	
hippopotamus	aspire	worst	xx
canvas	correspond	person	
	atmosphere	reversal	hoist
xx	hemisphere		moist
		nursery	moisten
	[ɝs]	personal	
damask	xx	personality	oyster
locust	butterscotch	mercenary	moisture

Vowel + [s] + Vowel (The vowel following [s] is noted.)

[si]

reseal
precede
recede
receive
deceit
deceive
beseech
besiege
Lucile
proceed
casino
panacea
intercede
oversea

[sɪ]

creasing
increasing
greasy
leasing
releasing
fleecing
hissing
kissing
prissy
precision
noticing
practicing
decision
menacing
harnessing
elicit
missing
missive
promising
racing
erasing
tracing
bracing
embracing
casing
lacy
lacing
placing
chasing
pacing
basic
facing
aggressive
dressing
pressing
depressing
impressive
guessing
blessing
message
confessing
icy
icing
icicle
tricycle
pricing
bicycle
acid
grassy
brassy
gassy
antacid
classic
classify
glassy
placid
passing
passage
massive
amassing
facet
prosecute
posse
crossing
tossing
glossy
bossy
mossy
faucet
engrossing
introducing
producing
lucid
elusive
juicy
fussy
assimilate
heresy
accuracy
piracy
courtesy
fantasy
jealousy
policy
fallacy
Pacific
pharmacy
deficit
facility
vicinity
cursing
cursive
nursing
persecute
reversing
conversing
voicing

[se]

resale
disable
essay
crusade
assay
assail
palisade
forsake
conversation

[sɛ]

reset
resell
precept
reception
deception
descent
descend
descendant
December
bisect
myself
asset
Yosemite
assent
assemble
assembly
procession
antiseptic
commissary
herself
percent
percentage

[saɪ]

recite
recital

		[sə]	
decide	massage	electricity	philosophy
beside	facade	disagree	glossary
wayside	[sɔ]	disadvantage	blossom
eyesight	disorder	disappear	possible
lucite	assorted	disappoint	impossible
aside	parasol	disapprove	possum
assign	basalt	discipline	animosity
asylum	[so]	admissible	gruesome
parasite	resold	recipe	cumbersome
Messiah	disown	decimal	anniversary
homicide	passover	acetate	
germicide	associate	casserole	[sɚ]
oversight	episode	taciturn	
underside	promissory	classify	oppressor
undersign	[su]	pacify	professor
	bassoon	capacity	ascertain
[sɑ]	assume	bassinet	
	[sʌ]	ambassador	[sɝ]
dishonor	honeysuckle	massacre	
disarm	asunder	ocelot	research
casaba		gossip	assert

25

Words Which May Be Difficult at the Beginning of Therapy

[s]—[s]

cease
seacoast
seesaw
seasick
seaside
serious
seersucker
six
sixty
sixteen
citrus
since
sincere
sinister
cyst
sister
system
sentence
centerpiece
sense
censor
sensation
sensible
cellulose
cesspool
semicircle
semblance
psychiatrist
sinus
silex
silence
cypress
sarcastic
solace
sauce
saucy
saucer
sausage

saucepan
source
soloist
sucrose
suitcase
sunset
suspect
substitute
somersault
suffix
cerise
succeed
success
solicit
celestial
society
sustain
suspect
suspend
suspicion
suggest
suppose
suppress
subscribe
subsist
semester
suffice
sophisticate
circumference
surpass
circus
circumstance
surplus
surface
service
space
spice
sparse

sports
spruce
splice
states
stamps
staffs
starts
stomps
stoops
stuffs
skates
scarce
slice
Swiss

abscess
absence
analysis
applesauce
armistice
asbestos
asparagus
assess
assist
asterisk
axis
basis
biceps
boisterous
crisscross
consequence
consist
conspicuous
crisis
diagnosis
discuss
disgrace
disgust

dishonest
distance
ecstasy
essence
excellence
excess
excuse
experience
express
hostess
hypnosis
incense
justice
license
listless
Mississippi
necessary
nuisance
persist
pessimist
phosphorous
precise
princess
process
recess
resource

[sks]

risks
frisks
disks
obelisks
whisks
desks
asks
casks
tasks
flasks

26

basks
masks
husks
rusks
tusks
dusks
damasks

[sts]

priests
beasts
feasts
wrists
jurists
forests
dentists
lists
mists
chemists
fists
harvests
tastes
pastes
bastes
wastes
rests
arrests
crests
guests
tests
detests
contests
nests
chests
jests
digests
pests

vests
invests
casts
lasts
blasts
masts
fasts
frosts
costs
hosts
roasts
coasts
ghosts
toasts
posts
boasts
roosts
rusts
crusts
trusts
gusts
dusts
adjusts
busts
combusts
ballasts
breakfasts
bursts
ousts
hoists

[sps]

crisps
lisps
wisps
asps
hasps
rasps

grasps
clasps
wasps

[z]–[s]

zest
disaster
exist
irresistible
possess
resist

[s]–[z]

seize
season
series
citizen
sizzle
civilize
centralize
selves
size
sizable
sarcasm
supervise
suds
sunrise
surprise
surmise

capsize
chastise
despise
disguise
downstairs
emphasize
excise
excuse

expose
incisor
italicize
masses
messes
Mrs.
molasses
pasteurize
upstairs

[snz]

christens
listens
glistens
hastens
basins
masons
lessons
bisons
fastens
loosens
moccasins
medicines
persons
moistens

[slz]

bristles
missiles
whistles
wrestles
trestles
nestles
vessels
castles

27

tassels
jostles
fossils
hustles
rustles
bustles
muscles
reversals

[s] — [θ]

sixth
sixteenth
synthetic
sympathy
seventh
seventeenth
psychopath
Sabbath
sooth
something
south
southeast
southeastern
southland
southpaw
southwest
stethoscope
strength
strengthen
sloth
sleuth
smith
smithy

esthetic
anesthetic

28

anesthetist
anesthesia
calisthenics

[θ] — [s]

thesis
thistle
thistledown
thespian
thefts
thymus
thanks
Thanksgiving
thankless
thoughts
thorax
thumbtacks
thumps
thirst
thirsty
thermos
threats
thrice
thrombosis
throats
thrust
thwarts

heaths
wreaths
Keith's
sheaths
faiths
breaths
deaths
laths
paths

baths
froths
cloths
moth's
oaths
growths
booths
earths
births
hearths
fourths
mouths
tenths
months
twelfths
fifths

arthritis
ruthless
bathhouse
birthplace
mouthpiece
hypothesis
parenthesis
afterthoughts
ethics
athletics
mathematics
toothpicks
toothaches
birthmarks
orthodox
amethyst
atheist
northeast
northwest
northernmost

bloodthirsty
anthracite

[s] — [ð]

seethe
soothe
southern
southerner
southerly
southernmost
scathe
stepbrother
stepmother
stepfather
slither
smithereens
smooth
smoother
smoothen
swarthy

trustworthy

[ð] — [s]

this
thence
thenceforth
thyself
that's
thus
themselves
thereabouts

farthest
furthest
withstand
loathsome
nevertheless

Z

[z]

Construction of the [z] Word Lists

1. There are four categories:
    a. the [z] followed by a vowel including initial [z] and medial [z] blends.
    b. the [z] preceded by a vowel including final [z] and final and medial [z] blends.
    c. the [z] preceded and followed by a vowel.
    d. final and medial [z] blends [r z, g z, ŋ z, d z, n z, l z, b z, m z, v z, ð z].

2. Where appropriate, the [z] is combined with other consonants in the order which follows:
    [h, j, r, k, g, ŋ, t, d, n, l, s, z, ʃ, ʒ, tʃ, dʒ, p, b, m, f, v, θ, ð, hw, w].
    The words zenith, zeal, zebra; or he's, keys, tease, knees, seize, cheese, peas, bees, these, and wheeze illustrate some of these combinations. If a slight shift in vowels is desired, words such as he's, his, haze, has, hose, whose, hers, and house are the first or second words in the lists because [h] is the first consonant combined with [z].

3. Where appropriate, the [z] is combined with vowels and diphthongs in the order which follows:
    [i, ɪ, e, ɛ, aɪ, æ, ɑ, ɔ, o, ʊ, u, ʌ, ə, ɚ, ɜ, ɝ, aʊ, ɔɪ, ju].

4. When there are two [z] sounds in a word, the second [z] is underlined.

5. To facilitate the location of words in a category, medial [z] words are noted by xx.

Characteristics and Use of the [z] Word Lists

1. Choose words which are appropriate for the age and interests of the client. Many words are listed for high school students and adults but would not be considered for small children. The lists also reflect the relative frequency of each vowel in combination with [z]. For example, there are many more words ending with [aɪ z] than [ɛ z].

29

2. Determine which sound combination is the easiest.
   a. If it is [z] + Vowel, begin on page 31. Choose the vowel which makes [z] production easiest.
   b. If it is Vowel + [z], begin on pages 32—34. Choose the vowel which makes [z] production easiest.
   c. If it is a final blend, begin with that blend on pages 36—39. Frequently the [dz, nz, lz] are easy.

3. It may or may not be desirable to proceed down the Vowel + [z] lists through the medial blends. If it is not, skip to the next list.

Methods of Correcting the [z] Sound

About half of the people produce the [z] sound with their tongue tip behind, but not touching, the upper central incisors and about half produce it by putting their tongue tip behind the lower central incisors. The tongue blade and alveolar ridge are used to make the [z]. The lower teeth must be clearly visible if a sharp, clear [z] sound is to be produced. The lower lip must be pulled down or the [z] will be fuzzy.

The auditory-visual method of teaching the [z] is preferred and should be attempted first. However, some clients are unable to say the [z] without additional assistance.

If a placement method is used, the tongue tip and alveolar ridge production of [z] usually should be attempted first because [z] frequently is combined with other tongue tip sounds [d, n, l] in words and conversation and less tongue adjustment is required if the [z] also is produced with the tongue tip. However, some clients find the tongue blade production of [z] much easier, particularly if they have a very wide alveolar ridge. If an acoustically acceptable [z] sound is produced, it is unimportant whether the tongue tip is up or down.

The [z] is the voiced cognate of the [s]. Therefore, the suggestions for the correction of the [s] sound, made on pages 2—5, would apply to the [z], except that in numbers 3 and 6 use the [d] instead of the [t] and in number 4 use [nd] and [ndz].

If the client can say the [s], you need only to indicate the addition of voice. If difficulty is encountered, ask the client to put his hand on your throat as you say [z] and then feel the vibration in his own throat as he says [z].

[z] + Vowel

[z i]

zee	zipper	czarina	Zeus
zenith	zither	zombi	zoom
zeal			
zebra	xx	[z o]	[z ə]
	clumsy		xx
xx	flimsy	zodiac	Kansas
benzene	frenzy	zone	stanza
		zoology	bonanza
[z ɪ]	[z ɛ]		influenza
zero	zealous	xx	
zigzag	zest		[z ɝ]
zing	zephyr	Alonzo	zircon
zinc			xx
zinnia	[z ɑ]	[z u]	observe
zip	czar	zoo	observatory

Vowel + [z] *

[iz]

ease	series	praise	presence
he's	Indies	appraise	pleasant
degrees	sixes	braise	pheasant
breeze	bases	defrays	Presbyterian
freeze	Mrs.	gaze	
keys	judges	agaze	## [aɪz]
skis	fizz	daze	
tease	whiz	mayonnaise	eyes
knees	always	glaze	rise
sneeze		blaze	arise
please	xx	ablaze	memorize
fleas		chaise	cries
seize	prison	crochets	tries
she's	imprison	maize	dries
cheese	isn't	amaze	sunrise
peas	drizzle	phase	prize
bees	frizzle	sideways	comprise
these	sizzle		fries
wheeze	chisel	xx	skies
squeeze	fizzle		guise
	dismal	brazen	disguise
xx		hazel	ties
	miserable	nasal	magnetize
reason	business		alphabetize
treason	prisoner	nasalize	dramatize
season	grizzly		advertise
easel	drizzly	## [ɛz]	baptize
	Lisbon		dies
cheesecake		says	iodize
cheesecloth	## [ez]	fez	standardize
easement			merchandise
beeswax	haze	xx	denies
	raze		organize
## [ɪz]	craze	embezzle	modernize
	graze		harmonize
is	trays	Ezra	
his		present	

---

*Words ending with ed are not listed. If [zd] blends are desired, ed may be added to many of the final [z] words listed above.

recognize
lies
realize
size
exercise
emphasize
publicize
shies
apologize
pies
spies
despise
buys
compromise
defies
supervise
revise
advise
wise

xx

horizon
reprisal

wisecrack

[æz]

as
has
razz
whereas
Alcatraz
jazz

xx

frazzle
dazzle

Aztec
asthma
hasn't
has-been
raspberry

[ɑz]

awes
was

xx

rosin
wasn't
nozzle
cosmic
cosmetic
cosmopolitan
Moslem

[ɔz]

draws
cause
because
gauze
laws
clause
applause
pause

xx

causeway

[oz]

owes
hose

rose
arose
crows
grows
prose
primrose
froze
echoes
goes
toes
tomatoes
potatoes
doze
bulldoze
nose
gallows
close
enclose
disclose
glows
flows
chose
pose
oppose
propose
repose
expose
dispose
compose
those

xx

frozen
chosen

nosegay
clothesline
clothespin

clothesbasket
nosebleed

[uz]

whose
cruise
bruise
snooze
lose
blues
choose

[juz]

use
accuse
excuse
dues
news
misuse
abuse
mews
amuse
fuse
refuse
confuse

xx

accusal
refusal

newsreel
newsstand
newspaper
newsprint
fuselage

33

[ʌz]

does
buzz
fuzz

xx

cousin
dozen
doesn't
guzzle
puzzle
muzzle

muslin
husband

[əz]

comas
commas

xx

artisan

inasmuch

[ɚz]

fingers
sisters
dinners
pliers
colors
scissors
bleachers
diapers
divers
rivers

[ɝz]

errs
hers

curs
stirs
slurs
blurs
sirs
shirrs
purrs
burrs
furs
firs

xx

Thursday

[auz]

house
rouse

xx

arouse
carouse

xx

tousle

[ɔɪz]

corduroys
noise
joys
poise
boys

xx

poison

34

Vowel + [z] + Vowel (The vowel following [z] is noted.)

[zi]

disease
magazine
museum

[zɪ]*

easy
freezing
teasing
sneezing
sleazy
resist
dizzy
busy
busily
visit
hazy
crazy
daisy
lazy
rising
advertising
closet
deposit
rosy
cozy
posy
closes
Moses
buzzing
fuzzy
position
opposite
Brazil
physician

frowsy
lousy
noisy
using
music
musician

[ze]

azalea
dramatization
organization

[zɛ]

resent
resemble

[zaɪ]

reside
resign
desire
desirable
design

[zæ]

disaster

[zɑ]

resolve
dissolve
horizontal
bazaar
Amazon

[zɔ]

resort

[zʊ]

Missouri

[zu]

resume
presume
Montezuma
Kalamazoo

[zʌ]

result

[zə]

Pisa
invisible
divisible
inquisitive
heroism
conservatism
journalism
realism
optimism
resident
president
residue
resolution
advisable
plaza
spasm
rosary
bosom

[zɝ]

Caesar
tweezers
gizzard
lizard
blizzard
scissors
wizard
razor
razorback
desert
kaiser
geyser
appetizer
miser
visor
divisor
adviser
hazard
cruiser
buzzard

[zɜ]

reserve
preserve
dessert
desertion
deserve

[zaʊ]

resound

---

*Only a few words ending with ing are listed. If additional words are desired, add ing to appropriate words in the Vowel + [z] section.

Final and Medial [z] Blends

[rz]

ears	choirs	pegs	gangs
hears	cars	begs	pangs
years	scars	rags	bangs
gears	cigars	gags	fangs
tears	guitars	tags	wrongs
steers	jars	nags	gongs
nears	spars	lags	tongs
shears	bars	sags	songs
cheers	mars	bags	
jeers	wars	wags	
piers	oars	hogs	## [dz]
appears	cores	cogs	
spears	doors	togs	reads
smears	ignores	jogs	creeds
fears	snores	bogs	deeds
heirs	explores	dogs	needs
cares	floors	logs	leads
scares	shores	rogues	pleads
tears	chores	hugs	seeds
stares	pours	rugs	beads
dares	bores	tugs	feeds
snares	tours	lugs	weeds
declares	insures	bugs	rids
glares	ours	mugs	kids
shares	hours		lids
chairs	scours		bids
pairs	sours	## [ŋz]	aids
spares	devours		raids
compares		rings	grades
bears		brings	degrades
mares	## [gz]	kings	trades
affairs		stings	fades
wears	rigs	sings	wades
squares	digs	pings	heads
hires	jigs	things	reds
tires	pigs	wings	sheds
admires	wigs	swings	weds
fires	eggs	savings	hides
wires	kegs	hangs	rides
	legs		

tides	winds	leans	moans
sides	ends	jeans	prunes
adds	tends	queens	tunes
comrades	lends	tins	moons
dads	sends	shins	guns
lads	spends	chins	tons
pads	bends	pins	sons
fads	mends	bins	puns
odds	rinds	fins	buns
gods	grinds	thins	
nods	kinds	wins	yarns
pods	binds	rains	barns
wads	minds	canes	horns
odes	finds	gains	corns
roads	hands	detains	acorns
codes	stands	lanes	scorns
toads	lands	complains	thorns
loads	glands	chains	warns
modes	sands	pains	mourns
floods		manes	
suds	yields	wanes	xx
crowds	fields	dines	
	builds	lines	Wednesday
	scalds	signs	
beards	holds	shines	[l z]
yards	scolds	pines	
cards	molds	mines	eels
discards	folds	fines	heels
guards	worlds	wines	reels
bards		cans	deals
cords	xx	tans	kneels
lords		pans	seals
wards	tradesman	bans	peals
hoards	bridesmaid	fans	meals
chords	bondsman	groans	feels
gourds		cones	wheels
towards	[n z]	tones	hills
swords		loans	kills
boards	teens	bones	gills
	deans		

37

sills	holes	fiddles	nabs
chills	rolls	cradles	labs
pills	souls	ladles	hobs
bills	poles	saddles	robs
mills	bowls	paddles	cobs
fills	moles	toddles	gobs
wills	foals	dawdles	knobs
hails	rules	waddles	sobs
rails	tools	noodles	jobs
gales	duels	poodles	mobs
tails	jewels	huddles	fobs
details	pools	puddles	robes
nails	fools		probes
snails	hulls	kindles	lobes
sails	gulls	handles	tubes
jails	oils	candles	hubs
pails	coils	scandals	rubs
bails	toils	sandals	grubs
males	soils	fondles	cubs
fails	spoils	bundles	tubs
whales	boils		dubs
tells	foils	xx	clubs
sells		salesman	
shells	snarles		garbs
bells	Charles	[bz]	barbs
wells		ribs	absorbs
tiles	whittles	cribs	
piles	nettles	bibs	[mz]
miles	settles	fibs	
files	petals	babes	Reims
gals	titles	debs	creams
dolls	rattles	webs	dreams
halls	tattles	tribes	teams
calls	battles	jibes	deems
shawls	bottles	crabs	seems
balls		grabs	beams
falls	needles	gabs	themes
walls	riddles	tabs	rims
	middles	dabs	trims

dims	dooms	beeves	loves
limbs	looms	thieves	gloves
gyms	hums	weaves	shoves
games	crumbs	gives	serves
tames	comes	lives	
flames	gums	sieves	carves
shames	sums	raves	starves
James	bums	craves	
hems	thumbs	graves	elves
gems		saves	delves
rhymes	arms	shaves	selves
crimes	harms	paves	shelves
times	alarms	waves	valves
dimes	charms	hives	solves
limes	farms	drives	wolves
climbs	storms	thrives	
chimes	forms	dives	
hams	informs	knives	xx
rams	warms	chives	
crams		fives	eavesdrop
trams	elms	wives	
drams	helms	halves	[ð z]
lambs	realms	calves	
jams		salves	wreathes
alms	xx	roves	breathes
calms		groves	teethes
psalms	Jamestown	coves	seethes
palms	doomsday	loaves	bathes
bombs		cloves	writhes
homes	[v z]	hooves	tithes
roams		grooves	loathes
domes	eaves	proves	soothes
foams	grieves	moves	truths
rooms	leaves	doves	smooths
	sleeves		
	peeves		

S

[ʃ]

[ʃ]

Construction of the [ʃ] *Word Lists*

1. There are four categories:
   a. the [ʃ] followed by a vowel including initial [ʃ] and medial [ʃ] blends.
   b. the [ʃ] preceded by a vowel including final [ʃ] and final and medial [ʃ] blends.
   c. the [ʃ] preceded and followed by a vowel.
   d. initial, medial, and final [ʃ] blends.

2. Where appropriate, the [ʃ] is combined with other consonants in the order which follows:

   [h, j, r, k, g, ŋ, t, d, n, l, s, z, ʃ, ʒ, tʃ, dʒ, p, b, m, f, v, θ, ð, hw, w].

   The words shuck, shut, shun, shush, shove; or hush, rush, gush, lush, and mush illustrate some of these combinations. If a slight shift in vowels is desired, words such as sheik, shake, shack, shock, shook, shuck, and shirk are found near the beginning of the lists because [k] is combined with [ʃ] after [h, j, r].

3. Where appropriate, the [ʃ] is combined with vowels and diphthongs in the order which follows:

   [i, ɪ, e, ɛ, aɪ, æ, ɑ, ɔ, o, ʊ, u, ʌ, ə, ɚ, ɜ, ʒ, aʊ, ɔɪ, ju].

4. When there are two [ʃ] sounds in a word, the second [ʃ] is underlined.

5. To facilitate the location of a word in a category, medial [ʃ] words are noted by xx and final [ʃ] blends are noted by xxx.

Characteristics and Use of the [ʃ] *Word Lists*

1. Choose words which are appropriate for the age and interests of the client. Many words are listed for high school students and adults but would not be considered for small children. The lists also reflect the relative frequency of each vowel in combination with [ʃ]. For example, there are many more words beginning with [ʃæ] than [ʃaʊ].

2. Determine which sound combination is the easiest.
   a. If it is [ʃ] + Vowel, begin on pages 44–46. Choose the vowel which makes the [ʃ] production easiest.
   b. If it is Vowel + [ʃ], begin on pages 47–48. Choose the vowel which makes the [ʃ] production easiest.

3. It may or may not be desirable to proceed down the [ʃ] + Vowel lists through the medial blends. If it is not desirable, skip to the next list.

Methods of Correcting the [ʃ] Sound

The [ʃ] is produced with the tongue blade and alveolar ridge. The tongue tip is usually behind, but not touching, the upper central incisors but a few children put their tongue tip behind their lower central incisors and produce an acoustically acceptable [ʃ] sound. The important aspects of [ʃ] production seem to be as follow:
   1. The breath stream is emitted centrally.
   2. The muscles at the corners of the mouth are tightened and press against the upper teeth.
   3. The lips are slightly puckered.
The auditory-visual method of teaching the [ʃ] is preferred and should be attempted first. However, in some cases, the client is unable to say the [ʃ] without additional assistance. The following ideas have been helpful in these instances.

1. Ask the client to place his forefinger on his nose and chin, vertically, and to touch his finger with his lips as he makes the hushing sound, [ʃ]. For small children, associate this action with a mother quieting the children when the baby is sleeping. Use a mirror to observe lip movement.

2. If the tongue is protruding on the [ʃ], ask the client to close his teeth as if he were chewing, pucker his lips, and blow.

3. If the [ʃ] is lateral and the [s] is made correctly, ask the client to prolong the [s] sound as you gently push the sides of his lips against his upper teeth with your thumb and forefinger. Gradually push the sides of the lips forward against the teeth until the lips pucker. This usually produces a sound somewhere between [s] and [ʃ] but, with practice, it is not hard to develop a good [ʃ] sound. If the client slips into a lateral [ʃ] as the lips move forward, stop immediately

and remind him to "think [s]." If difficulty is encountered when he tries the [ʃ] unassisted, ask him to look in a mirror and determine which of the three aspects of production, mentioned earlier, is faulty. Before using this method, check the production of the [s] with a drinking straw to be sure the breath is emitted centrally.* Occasionally, a client will produce an acoustically acceptable [s] which is emitted laterally. In these cases, teach central emission of the [s] before attempting to teach the [ʃ].

4. Ask the client to say [n]. Ask him to feel the contact of the tongue and gum ridge. Tell him to drop the tip of his tongue slightly without breaking the lateral contact and say [ʃ]. The [n] is used for position only. Do not ask the client to prolong the [n] and add the [ʃ] because the resulting sound is usually [ntʃ].

---

*Hold a drinking straw at a forty-five degree angle against the edges of the upper central incisors. As the client prolongs the [s] sound, move the straw along the edge of the teeth until the point of breath emission is located.

[ʃ] + Vowel*

[ʃi]

she	shipshape	unshaken	Cheyenne
sheik	shipboard	unshaven	shyly
chic	shipbuilder		Shylock
sheet	shipmate	**[ʃɛ]**	shyster
she'd	shim		
sheen	shimmer	share	**xx**
chignon	shimmy	shareholder	
she'll	chiffon	Sharon	outshine
Sheila	shift	sherry	sunshine
shield	shiver	sheriff	moonshine
she's	chivalry	shekel	
sheep		Shetland	**[ʃæ]**
sheaf	**xx**	shed	
sheaves		shell	shack
sheath	warship	shelter	shackle
sheathe	courtship	shellproof	shag
	midship	shelf	Shanghai
xx	internship	shellfish	shank
	makeshift	shelves	shatter
banshee		shepherd	chateau
windshield	**[ʃe]**	chef	shad
newssheet		Chevrolet	shadow
	shay	chevron	shan't
[ʃɪ]	shake		chandelier
	shaker	**xx**	shall
shear	shaky		chalet
sheer	Shakespeare	nutshell	shallow
shingle	shade	soft-shell	shalt
shin	shale	bloodshed	shasta
shinny	chaise	cockleshell	chapeau
Shinto	shape	clamshell	chaperon
shindig	shame	bombshell	shabby
shilling	shamefaced		sham
ship	shave	**[ʃaɪ]**	chamois
shipyard			shamrock
shipwreck	**xx**	shy	shampoo
shipload		shine	champagne
	nightshade	shiny	

*Words ending with s, ed, and ing are not listed but should be considered if additional words are needed.

44

shamble
shaft

xx

foreshadow
crankshaft
ramshackle

[ʃɑ]

shah
shark
chartreuse
sharp
shock
shot
shod
shoddy
shop
shopkeeper

xx

earshot
buckshot
bloodshot
gunshot
pawnshop
roughshod

[ʃɔ]

shaw
short
shorthand
shortcake
shortbread
shawl

xx

ricksha

[ʃo]

show
shore
shorn
showroom
showcase
shoat
showdown
shone
shown
shoal
shoulder
showboat
showman
chauffeur

xx

inshore
offshore

[ʃʊ]

sure
shook
sugar
should
shouldn't

xx

cocksure
unsure
insure
insurance

[ʃu]

shoe
shoot
shoelace
shoestring

shoeshop
shoebrush
shoemaker

xx

outshoot
horseshoe
six-shooter
offshoot

[ʃʌ]

shuck
shut
shutter
shut-in
shutdown
shuttle
shuttlecock
shudder
shun
shunt
shush
shuffle
shove
shovel

[ʃə]

charade
Chicago
chagrin
chenille
shenanigan
shellac
shillelagh

xx

partial
marshal

contortion
distortion
portion
proportion
diction
dictionary
restriction
friction
fiction
conviction
correction
direction
connection
election
collection
complexion
section
affection
perfection
infection
action
reaction
traction
satisfaction
destruction
construction
production
introduction
suction
luxury
auction
anxious
sanction
conjunction
function
tension
attention
intention

45

detention
potential
confidential
presidential
pension
mention
dimension
prevention
convention

financial
mansion
conscious
orthodontia
description
prescription
subscription
exception
deception

contraption
option

[ʃɝ]

shirk
shirt
shirtwaist
Sherlock

Sherman
sherbert

xx

nightshirt

[ʃaʊ]

shout
shower

Vowel + [ʃ] *

[iʃ]

leash
unleash

[ɪʃ]

cherish
parish
perish
Irish
garish
licorice
impoverish
flourish
nourish
skittish
fetish
dish
radish
horseradish
outlandish
blandish
brandish
modish
diminish
finish
Danish
replenish
Spanish
banish
garnish
tarnish
varnish
admonish
punish
burnish
furnish

relish
embellish
establish
polish
demolish
accomplish
Polish
foolish
publish
rubbish
furbish
squeamish
blemish
famish
skirmish
fish
crayfish
elfish
shellfish
whitefish
catfish
flatfish
blackfish
crawfish
codfish
starfish
goldfish
bluefish
sunfish
ravish
lavish
dervish
wish
swish
relinquish

vanquish
distinguish
anguish
whish

xx

dishcloth
lavishness
wishbone
nourishment
punishment
establishment
accomplishment
dishful
wishful

[ɛʃ]

fresh
afresh
refresh
thresh
flesh
horseflesh
mesh
enmesh

[æʃ]

ash
hash
rash
crash
trash
brash
cash
cache

gash
succotash
potash
mustache
dash
gnash
lash
clash
slash
flash
eyelash
goulash
backlash
unlash
whiplash
sash
mash
smash
bash
abash

xx

flashlight
cashbook
cashmere
bashful

[ɑʃ]

slosh
kibosh
wash
quash
squash
backwash

---

*Words ending with ed are not included and should be considered if [ʃt] blends are desired.

47

hogwash	bush	crush	slush
whitewash	ambush	bulrush	plush
swash		inrush	blush
	xx	brush	flush
xx	pushcart	hairbrush	mush
washroom	bushman	paintbrush	
swashbuckle		clothesbrush	xx
	[ʌʃ]	thrush	
[ʊʃ]	hush	gush	
push	rush	lush	mushroom

48

Vowel + [ʃ] + Vowel (The vowel following [ʃ] is noted.)

[ʃi]

machine	sashay	pressure	suspicion
garnishee	reshape	rasher	exhibition
	ashamed	haberdasher	ambition
		washer	mission

[ʃɪ]

[ʃɛ]

kosher | omission

bushy
mashie
cashier
Washington
freshet
initiative
appreciate
initiate
officiate
satiate
associate
negotiate
dishes*
fishes
wishes
distinguishes
appreciation
initiation
negotiation
reship
censorship
professorship
insatiable

dishevel
watershed

[ʃo]

ashore
seashore
threshold

[ʃʊ]

issue
tissue
assure
reassure
assurance

[ʃu]

cashew
snowshoe
parachute

[ʃʌ]

smashup

[ʃɚ]

fissure
fisher
kingfisher
glacier

[ʃɝ]

undershirt

[ʃə]

Patricia
militia
fuchsia
Russia
inertia
Michigan
Venetian
nutrition
electrician
pediatrician
petition
repetition
competition
dentition
edition
addition
tradition
condition
definition
recognition
position
opposition
composition
preposition
musician

permission
commission
admission
intermission
station
nation
session
succession
concession
possession
expression
impression
depression
freshen
profession
confession
passion
compassion
fashion
caution
precaution
ocean
notion
lotion
motion
emotion
commotion
devotion
pincushion
solution

[ʃe]

crochet
ricochet
cliché
sachet

*Not all words ending with es and ing are listed. These endings may be added to many of the Vowel + [ʃ] words listed on pages 47—48 if additional words are desired.

resolution	insertion	official	vicious
revolution	desertion	artificial	cautious
institution	exertion	special	atrocious
constitution	rational	social	luscious
substitution	irrational	crucial	bishop
prosecution	national	bushel	perishable
contribution	international	controversial	fashionable
distribution	nationality	facetious	washable
assertion	initial	delicious	sociable

Initial, Final, Medial [ʃ] Blends

shriek	shredded	shrunk	marshmallow
shrink	shrine	shrunken	enshrine
shrinkage	shrank	shrub	
shrill	shrapnel	shrubbery	
shrilled	shrove		
shrimp	shrew	xxx	
shrivel	shrewd		
shriveled	shrug	harsh	
shred	shrugged	marsh	

51

731C1

3

Construction of the [ʒ] *Word Lists*

1. There are three categories:
    a. the [ʒ] preceded by a vowel.
    b. the [ʒ] preceded and followed by a vowel.
    c. the [ʒ] followed by a vowel in a medial blend.

2. Where appropriate, the [ʒ] is combined with other consonants in the order which follows:

    [h, j, r, k, g, ŋ, t, d, n, l, s, z, ʃ, ʒ, tʃ, dʒ, p, b, m, f, v, θ, ð, hw, w].

3. Where appropriate, the [ʒ] is combined with vowels and diphthongs in the order which follows:

    [i, ɪ, e, ɛ, aɪ, æ, ɑ, ɔ, o, ʊ, u, ʌ, ə, ɚ, ɜ, ɝ, aʊ, ɔɪ, ju].

Characteristics and Use of the [ʒ] *Word Lists*

1. Few words with [ʒ] would be used with small children but they are listed for use with high school students and adults.

2. The words in the Vowel + [ʒ] lists will probably be easier than words in the Vowel + [ʒ] + Vowel lists.

Methods of Correcting the [ʒ] *Sound*

The [ʒ] is produced with the tongue blade and alveolar ridge. The tongue tip is usually behind, but not touching, the upper central incisors but a few children put their tongue tip behind their lower central incisors and produce an acoustically acceptable [ʒ] sound.

The [ʒ] is the voiced cognate of the [ʃ]. Therefore, the suggestions for the correction of the [ʃ] sound, made on pages 42–43, would apply to the [ʒ]. However, if the client can say the [ʃ] you need only to indicate the addition of voice. If difficulty is encountered, ask the client to put his hand on your throat as you say [ʒ] and then feel the vibration in his own throat as he says [ʒ].

Vowel + [ʒ]

[iʒ]	[ɑʒ]		[oʒ]
prestige	garage	fuselage	loge
	mirage	camouflage	
[eʒ]	entourage	corsage	[uʒ]
	sabotage	massage	
beige	ménage		rouge

Vowel + [ʒ] + Vowel (The vowel following [ʒ] is noted.)

[ʒi]

regime

[ʒɪ]

amnesia
Asiatic
fantasia
ambrosia

[ʒe]

negligee
protégé

[ʒʊ]

visual
visualize
casual

[ʒu]

bijou

[ʒə]

cohesion
adhesion
artesian
lesion
Parisian

derision
elision
collision
decision
precision
incision
vision
revision
division
provision
television
envision
Asia
abrasion
occasion
Caucasian
aphasia
evasion
invasion
persuasion
treasury
erosion
corrosion
explosion
intrusion
obtrusion

protrusion
contusion
allusion
collusion
delusion
disillusion
seclusion
inclusion
conclusion
exclusion
fusion
confusion
profusion
transfusion
excursion
Persia
Persian
aspersion
dispersion
emersion
version
aversion
conversion
diversion
inversion
subversion

usual
usually
unusual
usury
diffusion

[ʒɚ]

leisure
seizure
rasure
erasure
brazier
glazier
treasure
pleasure
measure
azure
crosier
crozier
closure
enclosure
inclosure
composure
disposure
exposure
Hoosier

Medial [ʒ] Blend

bourgeois

54

[tʃ]

Construction of the [tʃ] *Word Lists*

1. There are four categories:
    a. the [tʃ] followed by a vowel including initial [tʃ] and medial [tʃ] blends.
    b. the [tʃ] preceded by a vowel including final [tʃ] and medial [tʃ] blends.
    c. the [tʃ] preceded and followed by a vowel.
    d. final and medial [tʃ] blends [rtʃ, ntʃ, ltʃ].

2. Where appropriate, the [tʃ] is combined with other consonants in the order which follows:
    [h, j, r, k, g, ŋ, t, d, n, l, s, z, ʃ, ʒ, tʃ, dʒ, p, b, m, f, v, θ, ð, hw, w].
    The words cheer, cheek, cheat, cheese, cheap, chief; or reach, teach, leach, peach, and beach illustrate some of these combinations. If a slight shift in vowels is desired, words such as cheek, chick, check, chalk, choke, and chuck are found near the beginning of the lists because [k] is combined with [tʃ] after [h, j, r].

3. Where appropriate, the [tʃ] is combined with vowels and diphthongs in the following order:
    [i, ɪ, e, ɛ, aɪ, æ, ɑ, ɔ, o, ʊ, u, ʌ, ə, ɚ, ɜ, ɝ, aʊ, ɔɪ, ju].

4. When there are two [tʃ] sounds in a word, the second [tʃ] is underlined.

5. To facilitate the location of words in a category, medial [tʃ] words are noted by xx.

Characteristics and Use of the [tʃ] *Word Lists*

1. Choose words which are appropriate for the age and interests of the client. Many words are listed for high school students and adults but they would not be considered for small children. The lists also reflect the relative frequency of each vowel in combination with [tʃ]. For example, there are many more words beginning with [tʃɪ] than [tʃɔɪ].

55

2. Determine which sound combination is the easiest.
   a. If it is [tʃ] + Vowel, begin on pages 57—58. Choose the vowel which makes [tʃ] production easiest.
   b. If it is Vowel + [tʃ], begin on page 59. Choose the vowel which makes [tʃ] production easiest.
   c. If it is a final [tʃ] blend, begin with that blend on page 62.

3. It may or may not be desirable to proceed down the Vowel + [tʃ] lists through the medial blends. If it is not desirable, skip to the next list.

Methods of Correcting the [tʃ] *Sound*

The [tʃ] which is a combination of the [t] and the [ʃ] is usually produced with the tongue tip behind, but not touching, the upper central incisors but a few children put their tongue tip behind their lower central incisors and produce an acoustically acceptable [tʃ] sound.

The auditory-visual method of teaching the [tʃ] is preferred and should be attempted first. However, in some cases, the client is unable to say the [tʃ] without additional assistance. The ideas which follow have been helpful in these instances.

1. Explain to the client that [tʃ] is a combination of [t] and [ʃ]. Ask him to say [t] and then [ʃ]. Ask him to repeat these two sounds more and more rapidly until he says [tʃ].

2. If the tongue protrudes on the [tʃ], ask the client to close his teeth as if he were chewing and say [tʃ].

3. If the [tʃ] is lateral and the [ʃ] is made correctly, check production of the [t]. If the [t] also is made correctly, use the method described in number one above.

4. Ask the client to prolong the [n] sound and add [ʃ]. Ask him to make this sound combination stronger, louder, and faster. The resulting sound is usually [ntʃ]. Strengthen the sound by using the final [ntʃ] blends on page 62. The [l] may be used in the same manner to produce [ltʃ].

56

[tʃ] + Vowel*

[tʃ i]

cheer
cheerio
cheerily
cheerful
cheek
cheekbone
cheat
cheetah
cheese
cheesecake
cheesecloth
cheep
cheap
cheapen
chief

xx

Parcheesi
headcheese

[tʃ ɪ]

chick
chicory
chickadee
chicken
chicken pox
chickweed
chink
chit
chitchat
chin
chintz
chinchilla
chill
chilly

chili
children
chisel
chip
chipper
chipmunk
chimney
chimpanzee

xx

marching
mischief
benches
ranches
branches
lunches
bunches

[tʃ e]

chain
change
changeable
chase
chaste
chamber
chafe

xx

bedchamber
enchain
exchange

[tʃ ɛ]

chair

cherry
cherish
chairman
cherub
check
checker
checkerboard
checkroom
checkbook
checkmate
chess
chest
chestnut
chessboard
chessmen

xx

exchequer
hope chest
armchair

[tʃ aɪ]

chide
China
Chinese
child
childhood
childlike
chime

xx

godchild
grandchild
franchise
stepchild

[tʃ æ]

charity
charitable
chat
chatter
chatterbox
chattel
channel
chant
chance
challenge
chalice
chastise
chap
chapter
chapel
chaplain
champ
champion
chaff

xx

enchant
disenchant

[tʃ ɑ]

char
charcoal
chart
charter
chard
Charles
charge
charm
chock
chop

*Most words ending with es, ed, and ing are not included and should be considered if additional words are needed.

57

choppy
chop suey
chopstick

xx

discharge

[tʃɔ]

chaw
chortle
chalk
chocolate

[tʃo]

chore
choke
chokecherry
chose
chosen

xx

anchovy
rancho
poncho

[tʃʊ]
xx
mortuary
sanctuary
fluctuate

punctuate
intellectual
effectual
actual
contractual
tactual
factual
punctual
eventual
estuary
fistula

[tʃu]

chew
choose

[tʃʌ]

chuck
chuckle
chuck-full
chug
chunk
chutney
chub
chubby
chum
chummy
chump

[tʃə]
xx

Archibald
picturesque
structural
luncheon
cultural
celestial
congestion
digestion
suggestion
question
combustion

[tʃɚ]
x x

archer
departure
orchard
picture
lecture
conjecture
fracture
manufacture
structure
tincture
cincture
pinchers
denture
venture
adventure
cowpuncher
culture

pasture
posture
moisture
mixture
fixture
texture
scripture
rapture
capture
rupture
sculpture

[tʃɝ]

churn
churl
church
churchyard
chirp

[tʃɔr]

choice

[tʃau]

chow
chowder
chowchow
chow mein

Vowel + [tʃ] *

[itʃ]

each
reach
screech
outreach
preach
breach
breech
teach
leach
leech
bleach
beseech
peach
speech
impeach
beach

xx

beachcomber
peach tree
beach ball

[ɪtʃ]

itch
hitch
rich
enrich
stitch
cross-stitch
hemstitch
ditch
niche
snitch
pitch

which
witch
bewitch
twitch
sandwich
switch

xx

hitchhike
witchcraft
pitch-dark
pitchfork

[ɛtʃ]

retch
wretch
stretch
outstretch
homestretch
sketch
fetch
vetch

[ætʃ]

hatch
ratch
cratch
scratch
catch
detach
snatch
latch
unlatch

patch
crosspatch
dispatch
batch
match
mismatch

xx

scratch pad
detachment
matchmaker
catchword
patchwork

[ɑtʃ]

crotch
Scotch
butterscotch
hopscotch
splotch
blotch
botch
watch

xx

watchtower
watchdog
watchman
watchful

[otʃ]

roach
broach
brooch

reproach
coach
poach

xx

coachman

[ʌtʃ]

hutch
crutch
touch
retouch
Dutch
clutch
such
nonesuch
much

xx

touchdown

[ɝtʃ]

lurch
search
research
perch
birch

[aʊtʃ]

ouch
crouch
grouch
couch
slouch
pouch
vouch

*Words ending with ed are not listed but should be considered if practice on the [tʃt] blend is desired.

59

Vowel + [tʃ] + Vowel (The vowel following [tʃ] is noted.)

[tʃɪ]

reaching
preaching
teaching
reaches
screeches
preaches
teaches
peaches
speeches
beaches
itching
stitching
pitching
bewitching
switching
kitchen
kitchenette
kitchenware
itches
hitches
riches
stitches
ditches
pitches
witches
sandwiches
stretching
fetching
Gretchen
stretches
sketches
fetches
Apache
hatching
scratching
catching
snatching
patching
matching

hatchet
hatches
catches
detaches
patches
matches
watching
splotches
blotches
botches
watches
notching
notches
coaching
poaching
broaches
reproaches
coaches
poaches
touching
clutching
hutches
crutches
touches
clutches
kerchief
handkerchief
lurching
searching
lurches
searches
perches
birches
grouchy
crouching
slouching
crouches
grouches
slouches

pouches

[tʃe]

interchange

[tʃɛ]

highchair

[tʃæ]

bechance
perchance

[tʃɑ]

recharge
becharm
overcharge
surcharge

[tʃʊ]

obituary
habitual
ritual
situate
situation
spiritual
perpetuate
perpetual
statue
statute
statuesque
maturation
infatuate
literature
amateur
premature
virtue

virtual
mutual

[tʃə]

titular
witchery
treacherous
righteous
hatchery
natural
naturalize
saturate
satchel
bachelor
catchup
detachable
reproachable
approachable
escutcheon
merchandise

[tʃɚ]

creature
preacher
teacher
bleacher
feature
richer
miniature
furniture
pitcher
forfeiture
nature
denature
catcher

cowcatcher	butcher	signature	curvature
flycatcher	future	musculature	overture
stature	caricature	armature	nurture

Final and Medial [tʃ] Blends*

[r tʃ]

arch	lynch	bench	munch
starch	clinch	workbench	
cornstarch	flinch	wench	xx
parch	cinch	quench	
march	pinch	ranch	
scorch	finch	branch	pinch-hit
torch	goldfinch	avalanche	lunchroom
blowtorch	bullfinch	blanch	hunchback
	winch	haunch	henchman
xx	wrench	staunch	ranchman
archdeacon	trench	launch	
archduke	retrench	paunch	[l tʃ]
archduchess	intrench	hunch	
searchlight	entrench	crunch	milch
parchment	drench	scrunch	Welch
archway	French	lunch	squelch
	stench	punch	gulch
[n tʃ]	clench	bunch	mulch
inch			

*Words ending with ed are not included but should be considered if [tʃt] blends are desired.

62

d3

[dʒ]

[dʒ]

Construction of the [dʒ] *Word Lists*

1. There are four categories:
    a. the [dʒ] followed by a vowel including initial [dʒ] and medial [dʒ] blends.
    b. the [dʒ] preceded by a vowel including final [dʒ] and medial [dʒ] blends.
    c. the [dʒ] preceded and followed by a vowel.
    d. final and medial [dʒ] blends [rdʒ, ndʒ , ldʒ].

2. Where appropriate, the [dʒ] is combined with other consonants in the order which follows:
    [h, j, r, k, g, ŋ, t, d, n, l, s, z, ʃ, ʒ, tʃ, dʒ , p, b, m, f, v, θ, ð, hw, w].
    The words jade, Jane, jail, James; or rage, cage, guage, sage, page, and wage indicate some of these combinations. If a slight shift in vowels is desired, words such as Jean, Jane, John, Joan, June, and join are found near the middle of the lists because [dʒ] is combined with [n] after [ŋ, t, d].

3. Where appropriate, the [dʒ] is combined with vowels and diphthongs in the order which follows:
    [i, ɪ, e, ɛ, aɪ, æ, ɑ, ɔ, o, ʊ, u, ʌ, ə, ɚ, ɜ, ɝ, aʊ, ɔɪ, ju].

4. When there are two [dʒ] sounds in a word, the second [dʒ] is underlined.

5. To facilitate the location of words in a category, medial [dʒ] words are noted by xx.

Characteristics and Use of the [dʒ] *Word Lists*

1. Choose words which are appropriate for the age and interests of the client. Many words are listed for high school students and adults but would not be considered for small children. The lists also reflect the relative frequency of each vowel in combination with [dʒ]. For example, there are many more words beginning with [dʒɛ] than [dʒaʊ].

63

2. Determine which sound combination is the easiest.
   a. If it is [dʒ] + Vowel, begin on pages 65–67. Choose the vowel which makes [dʒ] production easiest.
   b. If it is Vowel + [dʒ], begin on pages 68–69. Choose the vowel which makes [dʒ] production easiest.
   c. If it is a final [dʒ] blend, begin with that blend on page 72.

3. It may or may not be desirable to proceed down the Vowel + [dʒ] lists through the medial blends. If it is not, skip to the next list.

Methods of Correcting the [dʒ] *Sound*

The [dʒ], which is a combination of the [d] and [ʒ], is usually produced with the tongue tip behind, but not touching, the upper central incisors but a few children put their tongue tip behind their lower central incisors and produce an acoustically acceptable [dʒ] sound.

The auditory-visual method of teaching [dʒ] is preferred and should be attempted first. However, in some cases, the client is unable to say the [dʒ] without additional assistance. The following ideas have been helpful in these instances.

The [dʒ] is the voiced cognate of the [tʃ]. If the client can say the [tʃ], you only need to indicate the addition of voice. If difficulty is encountered, ask the client to put his hand on your throat as you say [dʒ] and then feel the vibration in his own throat as he says [dʒ].

1. Explain to the client that [dʒ] is a combination of [d] and [ʒ]. Ask him to say [d] and then [ʒ]. Ask him to repeat these two sounds more and more rapidly until he says [dʒ].

2. If the tongue protrudes on the [dʒ], ask the client to close his teeth, as if he were chewing, and say [dʒ].

3. If the [dʒ] is lateral and the [ʒ] is made correctly, check production of the [d]. If the [d] also is made correctly, use the method described in number one above.

4. Ask the client to prolong the [n] sound and add [ʒ]. Ask him to make this sound combination stronger, louder, and faster. The resulting sound is usually [ndʒ]. Strengthen the sound by using the final [ndʒ] blends on page 72. The [l] may be used in the same manner to produce [ldʒ].

64

[dʒ] + Vowel*

[dʒi]

gee
geography
geology
geometry
gene
Jean
genie
genius
genial
genealogy
Jesus

xx

ingenious
meninges
pongee

[dʒɪ]

jeer
jig
jigger
jiggle
jigsaw
jingle
jitters
jitney
ginger
Jill
jilt
gip
gipsy
jib
giblet
gym
jimmy
jiffy

xx

margin
marginal
orgy
arranges
rangy
dingy
Algeria
bulges
divulges
discharges
subject

[dʒe]

jay
jayhawk
jaywalk
Jacob
jade
Jane
jail
jailbird
James

[dʒɛ]

Jerry
jet
jetty
jettison
jetsam
general
generalize
generally
generate
generous

genetic
gent
gentle
gentleman
gender
genuine
gel
jelly
gelatin
jealous
jealousy
jess
jest
gesture
jeopardy
jeopardize
gem
Gemini
Jeffrey

xx

suggest
suggestion
inject
injection
engender
ingest
angelic
evangelic
conjecture
congest
congestion
object
objection
objective

[dʒaɪ]

gyrate
gigantic
giant
jibe
gibe

xx

meningitis
angina

[dʒæ]

Jack
jacket
jackal
jackass
jack-in-the-box
jack-o'-lantern
jackrabbit
jackknife
jackstraw
jag
jaguar
jangle
Janet
janitor
Janice
jazz
jasmine
Japanese
jab
jabber
jam
jamb

*Words ending with s, ed, and ing are not listed.

[dʒʊ]

jamboree
javelin

xx

windjammer

[dʒɑ]

jar
jargon
jockey
jog
joggle
jot
John
jolly
jostle
job

[dʒɔ]

jaunt
jaundice
jawbone
jawbreaker

[dʒo]

Joe
joke
Joan
jolt
Joseph
jove
jovial

xx

banjo

jury
jurist
juror

xx

conjure
conjugal

[dʒu]

jewel
jute
Judy
Judith
judicial
June
juniper
julienne
July
Julia
Juliet
juice
jujutsu
jubilee
jubilation
jubilance
juvenile

[dʒʌ]

jug
juggle
jugular
junk
junket
junction
juncture
jungle

jut
just
justice
justify
judge
judgment
jump
jumbo
jumble

xx

conjunction
unjust
unjustified
injustice
misjudge

[dʒe]

giraffe
Jerusalem
jalopy
Japan

xx

Marjorie
margarine
sergeant
Argentina
Georgia
cordial
tangerine
longitude
dungeon
engine
engineer
astringent
tangent

pungent
ingenuity
vengeance
angel
Angelus
evangelize
changeable
tangible
intangible
algebra
algebraic
indulgence
divulgence

[dʒɚ]
xx

forger
injure
ginger
derringer
ranger
stranger
danger
endanger
manger
passenger
messenger
soldier

[dʒɝ]

jerk
jerkin
journey
journal
journalist
journalism
Jersey
germ

	[dʒɔɪ]	xx	[dʒaʊ]
German	joy	enjoy	jowl
Germany	join	enjoin	jounce
germinate	joint	disjoin	joust
germicide	Joyce	disjoint	
germane	joist		

Vowel + [dʒ] *

[idʒ]

liege
siege
besiege

[ɪdʒ]

voyage
ridge
carriage
courage
encourage
discourage
brokerage
storage
porridge
disparage
marriage
hemorrhage
forage
average
beverage
cartridge
partridge
bridge
abridge
drawbridge
suffrage
breakage
linkage
luggage
baggage
mortgage
heritage
cottage
vantage
advantage
disadvantage

percentage
vintage
hostage
vestige
wastage
adage
bandage
appendage
patronage
tonnage
lineage
personage
manage
mismanage
carnage
cartilage
pillage
village
college
knowledge
silage
foliage
message
passage
sausage
dosage
usage
envisage
cribbage
cabbage
herbage
garbage
midge
image
scrimmage
pilgrimage

damage
homage
plumage
rummage
cleavage
ravage
savage
salvage
language

xx

ridgepole
bridgework
encouragement
management
passageway

[edʒ]

age
rage
outrage
enrage
overage
cage
encage
gage
gauge
engage
disengage
stage
backstage
downstage
upstage
teen-age
sage

page
rampage
wage

xx

stagecoach
ageless
agelong
pageboy
engagement

[ɛdʒ]

edge
hedge
dredge
allege
sledge
pledge
fledge
wedge

xx

hedgehog
vegetable
fledgling
edgeways

[aɪdʒ]

oblige
disoblige

[ædʒ]

badge

---

*Words ending with ed are not listed and should be considered if [dʒd] blends are desired.

[ɑdʒ]

dodge   sludge
lodge   judge
hodgepodge   budge
               smudge
[ʌdʒ]   fudge
grudge
begrudge   xx
trudge
drudge   judgement

[ɝdʒ]

urge   verge
scourge
splurge   [judʒ]
dirge
serge   huge
surge   deluge
purge   refuge
merge
submerge

Vowel + [dʒ] + Vowel (The vowel following [dʒ] is noted.)

[dʒi]

squeegee
hygiene
Eugene

[dʒɪ] *

strategic
collegiate
Bridget
midget
rigid
frigid
aged
Reginald
register
registration
legislation
tragic
magic
gadget
imagine
imagination
majesty
magistrate
stodgy
podgy
logic
logical
pedagogy
pugilist
pugilistic
pudgy
budget

strategy
prodigy
elegy
trilogy
eulogy
neurology
psychology
otology
etiology
ideology
criminology
genealogy
physiology
zoology
sociology
geology
anthropology
biology
etymology
pathology
mythology
effigy
drudgery
origin
agility
magician
energy
allergy
clergy
perjury
allergic
surgical
virgin
Virginia

deluges

[dʒe]

bluejay

[dʒɛ]

eject
ejection
reject
rejection
deject
regenerate
degenerate
hygienic
digest
digestion
digestible
project
projectile
apologetic
photogenic
magenta
majestic
indigestible
eugenic

[dʒaɪ]

eulogize
apologize
energize

[dʒæ]

ejaculation
Ajax
highjacker
bluejacket
crackerjack
lumberjack

[dʒɑ]

ajar

[dʒɔ]

majority

[dʒu]

rejuvenate
rejuvenation

[dʒʌ]

prejudge
adjunct
adjust
maladjusted

[dʒə]

region
regional
regent
regency
legion
collegian
allegiance
Norwegian
refrigerate
refrigerator
religion
original

---

*The es and ing endings may be added to Vowel + [dʒ] words if additional words are needed.

originate	credulous	homogenize	manager
pigeon	incredulous	cogent	major
pigeonhole	legible	fugitive	ledger
pigeon-toed	illegible	cudgel	badger
vigil	regiment	bludgeon	codger
vigilant	regimental	oxygen	dodger
incorrigible	exaggerate	nitrogen	astrologer
eligible	exaggeration	hydrogen	dowager
plagiarize	menagerie	indigent	merger
contagion	agitate	intelligent	perjure
agency	agitator	intelligence	perjury
courageous	agitation	diligence	
outrageous	coadjutor	corrigible	[dʒɜ]
advantageous	tragedy	dirigible	adjourn
educate	pageant	sugery	sojourn
educator	imagination	surgeon	
education	agile	sturgeon	[dʒɔɪ]
vegetate	fragile	detergent	
vegetation	cogitate	insurgent	overjoy
prejudicial	cogitation	divergent	rejoin
legend	progeny	emergency	rejoice

Final and Medial [dʒ] Blends

[rdʒ]

large
charge
recharge
discharge
barge
gorge
engorge
George
forge

xx

bargemen

[ndʒ]

hinge
unhinge
orange
astringe
fringe
tinge
singe
lozenge
pinge
scavenge
twinge
range
arrange

disarrange
prearrange
derange
grange
strange
estrange
change
interchange
mange
avenge
revenge
flange
lunge

plunge
sponge
scrounge
lounge

xx

vengeful

[ldʒ]

bilge
indulge
bulge
divulge

θ

[θ]

[θ]

Construction of the [θ] *Word Lists*

1. There are four categories:
   a. the [θ] followed by a vowel including initial [θ] and medial [θ] blends.
   b. the [θ] preceded by a vowel including final [θ] and medial [θ] blends.
   c. the [θ] preceded and followed by a vowel.
   d. initial, medial, and final [θ] blends.

2. Where appropriate, the [θ] is combined with other consonants in the order which follows:
   [h, j, r, k, g, ŋ, t, d, n, l, s, z, ʃ, ʒ, tʃ, dʒ, p, b, m, f, v, θ, ð, hw, w].
   The words thick, thing, thin, thimble, thither; or kith, eightieth, Meridith, Kenneth, neolith, pith, and myth illustrate some of these combinations. If a slight shift in vowels is desired, words such as myth, math, moth, mirth, and mouth are found in the last half of the lists because [θ] is combined with [m] after [tʃ, dʒ, p, b].

3. Where appropriate, the [θ] is combined with vowels and diphthongs in the order which follows:
   [i, ɪ, e, ɛ, aɪ, æ, ɑ, ɔ, o, ʊ, u, ʌ, ə, ɚ, ɜ, ɝ, aʊ, ɔɪ, ju].

4. When there are two [θ] sounds in a word, the second [θ] is underlined.

5. To facilitate the location of words in a category, medial [θ] words are noted by xx and final [θ] blends are noted by xxx.

Characteristics and Use of the [θ] *Word Lists*

1. Choose words which are appropriate for the age and interests of the client. Many words are listed for high school students and adults but they would not be considered for small children. The lists also reflect the relative frequency of each vowel in combination with [θ]. For example, there are many more words beginning with [θi] than [θe].

73

2. Determine which sound combination is the easiest.
   a. If it is $[\theta]$ + Vowel, begin on page 75. Choose the vowel which makes $[\theta]$ production easiest.
   b. If it is Vowel + $[\theta]$, begin on pages 76—77.
   c. If it is a final $[\theta]$ blend, begin with that blend on page 79.

3. It may or may not be advisable to proceed down the $[\theta]$ + Vowel lists through the medial blends. If it is not, skip to the next list.

Methods of Correcting the $[\theta]$ Sound

   The auditory-visual method of teaching the $[\theta]$ is preferred and should be attempted first. However, in some cases, the client is unable to say the $[\theta]$ without additional assistance. The ideas which follow have been helpful in these instances.

1. Ask the client to bite the tip of his tongue lightly and blow. Use a mirror to observe tongue placement. For small children, this may be associated with a sandwich with the upper and lower teeth representing the bread and the tongue representing the sandwich filling.

2. Ask the client to say $[n]$, then to slide the tip of his tongue down the posterior portion of the upper central incisors until it protrudes, and blow. The $[l]$ may be used in the same manner. It must be recognized that both $[n]$ and $[l]$ are voiced while the $[\theta]$ is not. However, the instruction, "blow," usually produces a voiceless sound.

3. If the client substitutes $[f]$ for $[\theta]$, it may be necessary to inhibit the movement of the lower lip. Place a tongue depressor crosswise on the lower lip or place your thumb on the cleft of the chin and your forefinger under the chin and squeeze gently. The latter suggestion is not actually inhibitory but serves as a reminder to the client for self inhibition of lip movement. Use a mirror to monitor lip movement.

4. If the client substitutes $[t]$ for $[\theta]$ and is unable to produce $[\theta]$ by any of the above methods, ask him to say $[f]$. Ask him to listen to the sound and look in a mirror to observe placement. Ask him to use the tip of his tongue instead of his lower lip to make the $[f]$ sound. The result will be $[\theta]$.

[θ] + Vowel*

[θi]

theory
theoretic
theorize
theorem
theatrical
theater
Theodore
theology
theologian
theistic
thesis
theme
thematic
thief
thieve

xx

northeast
anaesthesia

[θɪ]

thick
thicket
thicken
thing
think
thin
thistle
thistledown
thimble
thither

xx

lengthy
filthy
healthy

wealthy
something
diphtheria

[θe]

theta

[θɛ]

therapy
therapeutic
thespian
theft

xx

synthetic
aesthetic
anaesthetics
calisthenics

[θaɪ]

thigh
thyroid
thymus

[θæ]

thank
thankless
Thanksgiving
thankful
thatch

[θɔ]

thaw
thorn

thong
thought

xx

forethought
afterthought
diphthong

[θo]

thorax

xx

menthol

[θu]

xx

enthuse
enthusiasm
enthusiastic

[θʌ]

thug
thud
thunder
thunderous
thunderhead
thundercloud
thunderstorm
thunderstruck
thumb
thumbtack
thumbnail
thump

[θə]

xx

Martha

orthodontic
orthodox
orthopedic
lengthen
Anthony
anthem
parenthesis
mentholated
anaesthetist
naphtha

[θɚ]

xx

Arthur
panther

[θɝ]

thorough
thirty
thirteen
third
thirst
thirsty
Thursday
thermos
thermostat
thermometer

[θaʊ]

thousand

*Words ending with s, ed, and ing are not listed.

Vowel + [θ]*

[iθ]

heath
wreath
Keith
teeth
beneath
underneath
sheath

[ɪθ]

kith
eightieth
fortieth
thirtieth
sixtieth
seventieth
nintieth
twentieth
fiftieth
Meredith
Kenneth
zenith
neolith
pith
myth
smith
goldsmith

xx

arithmetic

[eθ]

faith

xx

faithless
faithful

[εθ]

breath
death
Seth

xx

ethnic
Bethlehem
deathbed

[æθ]

hath
wrath
lath
path
bath
math
aftermath

xx

bathhouse
Catherine
bathroom
bathtub
athlete
athletic
Kathleen

pathfinder
lathwork
pathway

[ɑθ]

swath

[ɔθ]

betroth
broth
froth
cloth
tablecloth
cheesecloth
moth

xx

mothball

[oθ]

oath
growth
undergrowth
outgrowth
loath
sloth
both
quoth

[uθ]

youth
Ruth
truth

couth
uncouth
tooth
eyetooth
sleuth
sooth
forsooth
booth
vermouth

xx

Lutheran
ruthless
toothpick
toothpaste
toothbrush
truthful

[əθ]

Sabbath
Elizabeth
Plymouth

[ɝθ]

earth
dearth
unearth
birth
berth
rebirth
childbirth
mirth
worth

---

*Words ending with s and ed are not listed but should be considered if [θs, θt] blends are wanted.

76

xx   [aʊ θ]

birthright   birthplace   south   southpaw
earthquake   earthborn   mouth   mouthpiece
birthday   earthbound   cottonmouth   mouthful
earthly   birthmark   xx   southwest
worthless   earthworm   southland   southward

Vowel + [θ] + Vowel (The vowel following [θ] is noted.)

[θi]

amphitheater
cathedral
Athena
southeast
southeaster

[θɪ]

Ethiopia
everything
anything
smithy
mythical
within
atheist
plaything
ethical
ethics
Athens
Gothic
mothy
nothing
sympathy

[θe]

methane
Cathay
toothache

[θɛ]

authentic
psychotherapy
Othello
pathetic
hypothetic

[θɑ]

lethargic
lithographer
mythology
mythologist
pathos
python
pathology

pathologist
marathon
catholicism
methodic

[θɔ]

wherewithal
authority

[θə]

lethal
Elizabethan
Ithaca
lithograph
lithographic
Nathan
ethyl
Ethel
methyl
methylene

method
Methodist
stethoscope
Catholic
pathologic
mathematics
hypothesis
hypothesize
earthen
earthenware
Bertha

[θɚ]

ether
lethargy
author
authoress
authorize
Luther

Initial, Medial, and Final [θ] Blends

xx

three	thwart	lengthways	labyrinth
threesome			tenth
threescore	xxx	xxx	ninth
threefold			month
thrill	hearth	eighth	eleventh
thrift	north	heighth	seventh
thrifty	fourth		millionth
threat	swarth		
threaten		xx	xx
thread	xx		
thresh		cutthroat	enthrone
threshold	arthritic		enthrall
thrice	arthritis	xxx	anthracite
thrive	hearthstone		anthropology
thrash	forthright	width	monthly
throttle	forthcoming	breadth	
throb	North Carolina	hundredth	xxx
thrombosis	North Dakota	thousandth	
throng	northland		health
throw	northward	eighteenth	wealth
throat	northwest	nineteenth	filth
throne	forthwith	sixteenth	sixth
threw		seventeenth	depth
through	xxx	fourteenth	warmth
thrust	length	fifteenth	fifth
thrush	strength	thirteenth	twelfth

8

[ð]

$$[\eth]$$

Construction of the $[\eth]$ *Word Lists*

1. There are three categories:
    a. the $[\eth]$ followed by a vowel including initial $[\eth]$ and medial $[\eth]$ blends.
    b. the $[\eth]$ preceded by a vowel including final $[\eth]$ and medial $[\eth]$ blends.
    c. the $[\eth]$ preceded and followed by a vowel.

2. Where appropriate, the $[\eth]$ is combined with other consonants in the order which follows:
    $[h, j, r, k, g, \eta, t, d, n, l, s, z, \int, 3, t\int, d3, p, b, m, f, v, \theta, \eth, hw, w]$.
    The words they're, they'd, they'll, they've; or scathe, lathe, bathe, and swathe illustrate some of these combinations.

3. Where appropriate, the $[\eth]$ is combined with vowels and diphthongs in the order which follows:
    $[i, \textbf{I}, e, \varepsilon, a\textsc{i}, æ, \textscripta, \textopeno, o, \upsilon, u, \Lambda, \textschwa, \textrhookschwa, 3, \textrhookrevepsilon, a\upsilon, \textopeno\textsc{i}, ju]$.

4. When there is also a $[\theta]$ in the word, it is underlined.

5. To facilitate the location of words in a category, medial $[\eth]$ words are noted by xx.

Characteristics and Use of the $[\eth]$ *Word Lists*

1. Choose words which are appropriate for the age and interests of the client. Many words are listed for high school students and adults but they would not be considered for small children. The lists also reflect the relative frequency of each vowel in combination with $[\eth]$. For example, there are more words beginning with $[\eth\varepsilon]$ than $[\eth\textschwa]$.

2. Determine which sound combination is the easiest.
    a. If it is $[\eth]$ + Vowel, begin on page 83. Choose the vowel which makes $[\eth]$ production easiest.
    b. If it is Vowel + $[\eth]$, begin on page 84. Choose the vowel which makes $[\eth]$ production easiest.

3. It may or may not be advisable to proceed down the $[\eth]$ + Vowel lists through the medial blends. If it is not desirable, skip to the next list.

Methods of Correcting the $[\eth]$ Sound

The $[\eth]$ is the voiced cognate of the $[\theta]$. Therefore, the suggestions for the correction of the $[\theta]$ sound made on page 74 would apply to the $[\eth]$. However, if the client can say the $[\theta]$, you need only to indicate the addition of voice. If difficulty is encountered, ask the client to put his hand on your throat as you say $[\eth]$ and then feel his own throat as he says $[\eth]$.

[ð] + Vowel

[ði]

thee
these

xx

swarthy

[ðɪ]

this

xx

farthing
farthest

[ðe]

they
they're

they'd
they'll
they've

[ðɛ]

their
there
there's
therein
thereon
thereunder
thereupon
thereof
thereto
thereby
thereafter

therefore
then
thence
thenceforth
them
themselves

[ðaɪ]

thy
thyself
thine

[ðæ]

that
than

[ðo]

though
those

xx

although

[ðʌ]

thus

[ðə]

the

[ðɚ]

xx

northern
farther

[ðaʊ]

thou

Vowel + [ð] *

[ið]

wreathe
enwreathe
breathe
teethe
seethe
sheathe

[ɪð]

with
herewith
forthwith
wherewith

xx

rhythmic

withdraw
withdrew
withstand

[eð]

scathe
lathe
bathe
swathe

[ɛð]

xx

brethren

[aɪð]

writhe
tithe
blithe
scythe

[ɔð]

xx

moths

[oð]

loathe
clothe
unclothe

xx

loathsome
loathful

[uð]

soothe
smooth

xx

smoothness
smoothly

---

*Most words ending with ed and s are not listed. If [ðd] and [ðz] blends are desired, the endings may be added to many of the words listed above.

84

Vowel + [ð] + Vowel (The vowel following [ð] is noted.)

[ðɪ]

breathing
teething
seething
sheathing
bathing
writhing
tithing
clothing
soothing
furthest
worthy
trustworthy

[ðə]

heathen
rhythm
smithereens
leatherette
feathery
fathom

smoothen
nevertheless

[ðɚ]

either
neither
hither
hitherto
dither
slither
zither
smithers
thither
whither
wither
heather
together
tether
Netherlands
leather

feather
featherweight
pinfeather
weather
weathercock
weatherproof
rather
gather
lather
bother
father
fatherland
forefather
godfather
grandfather
stepfather
smoother
other
otherwise
brother
brotherhood

brotherly
stepbrother
another
southern
southerner
southernmost
southerly
mother
motherland
godmother
grandmother
stepmother
smother
further
furthermore

[ðaʊ]

without

[l]

Construction of the [l] Word Lists

1. There are four categories:
   a. the [l] followed by a vowel including initial [l] and initial and medial [l] blends [kl, gl, sl, pl, bl, fl] in that order.
   b. the [l] preceded by a vowel including final [l] and final and medial [l] blends.
   c. the [l] preceded and followed by a vowel.
   d. final and medial [l] blends [rl, kl, gl, tl, dl, nl, sl, zl, pl, bl, ml, fl, vl] and associated triple blends.
2. Where appropriate, the [l] is combined with other consonants in the order which follows:
   [h, j, r, k, g, ŋ, t, d, n, l, s, z, ʃ, ʒ, tʃ, dʒ, p, b, m, f, v, θ, ð, hw, w].
   The words lea<u>k</u>, lea<u>g</u>ue, lea<u>d</u>, lea<u>n</u>, lea<u>s</u>e, lea<u>sh</u>; or <u>h</u>eal, <u>r</u>eal, <u>k</u>eel, <u>t</u>eal, <u>d</u>eal, and <u>kn</u>eel illustrate some of the combinations. If a slight shift in vowels is desired, words such as l<u>ea</u>k, l<u>i</u>ck, l<u>a</u>ke, l<u>i</u>ke, l<u>a</u>ck, l<u>o</u>ck, l<u>oo</u>k, l<u>u</u>ck, and l<u>u</u>rk are found near the beginning of each list because [k] is combined with [l] after [h, j, r].
3. Where appropriate, the [l] is combined with vowels and diphthongs in the order which follows:
   [i, ɪ, e, ɛ, aɪ, æ, ɑ, ɔ, o, ʊ, u, ʌ, ə, ɚ, ɜ, ɝ, aʊ, ɔɪ, ju].
4. When there are two [l] sounds in the word, the second [l] is underlined.
5. To facilitate the location of words in a category, initial [l] blends are noted by x and medial [l] words are noted by xx.

Characteristics and Use of the [l] Word Lists

1. Choose words which are appropriate for the age and interests of the client. Many words are listed for high school students and adults but they would not be considered for small children. The lists also reflect the relative frequency of each vowel in combination with [l]. For example, there are many more words beginning with [lɪ] than [lɔr].
2. Determine which sound combination is the easiest.
   a. If it is [l] + Vowel, begin with that vowel on pages 90–95.
   b. If it is a Vowel + [l], begin with that vowel on pages 96–101.
   c. If it is a blend, begin with that blend on pages 90–95.
3. The initial and medial [l] blends are listed under initial [l] words in the [l] + Vowel section because the vowel influences the blend.

Proceed down the lists through the blends or skip to other initial [l] words and then come back to the blends. If the blends are taught later, a number of [gl] blends, for example, are easily found because the [gl] blends follow the [kl] blends in each list.

Methods of Correcting the [l] Sound

The [l] sound is usually produced with the tip of the tongue but a fairly large number of children produce an acoustically acceptable [l] with the tongue blade.

The auditory-visual method of teaching the [l] is preferred and is usually successful because the movement of the tongue is visible. However, in some cases, the client is unable to say the [l] without additional assistance. The ideas presented below have been helpful in these instances.

1. Many children learn to say [la] or [lɔ] rather easily. Strengthen it by using the [l] + Vowel to "sing" familiar songs such as *Happy Birthday to You* before proceeding to words in the [la] or [lɔ] lists.

2. Ask the client to open his mouth fairly wide. (Sometimes it is necessary to stabilize the jaw with a narrow tongue depressor on edge between the molars.) Stroke the alveolar ridge with a tongue depressor and ask him to touch the stroked area with his tongue tip as he says [la]. Have the client observe tongue movement in a mirror.

3. If further assistance is needed, stroke the alveolar ridge and the tongue tip with a tongue depressor. Ask the client to put the two stroked areas together as he says [la]. At first, it may be necessary to assist the tongue elevation with a tongue depressor.

4. If the client has difficulty raising his tongue tip voluntarily, ask him to say [da, ta] or [na] to determine whether or not he is capable of making the movement. If he can say these sounds, tell him that the [la] is said in almost the same way. If it is necessary to practice the above sounds to establish movement, use only the [d, t]. If the [n] is used, it may precipitate a nasal [l].

5. Demonstrate the movement of the tongue by extending your hand and raising your fingers for [ɔl] or dropping your fingers from the [l] position for [la]. Ask the client to say the sounds as you demonstrate.

88

6.   If the client substitutes [w/l] in [l] + Vowel words, use a mirror and call attention to the lip movement or inhibit lip movement by pushing the upper lip against the upper teeth with your thumb and forefinger.

7.   When teaching [kl, gl, pl, bl] blends, ask the client to place his tongue in the [l] position before saying the [k, g, p, b]. Or ask him to say an initial [l] word similar to the blend and then say the blend, for example, *loud-cloud, lad-glad, lay-play, Lou-blue.*

8.   For clients who distort the [l] by producing it with the back of the tongue and the soft palate, Vowel + [l] words are usually easier, particularly if the vowel requires the back of the tongue to be down as in [ɑ] or [ɔ]. Vowel + [l] + Vowel words are usually not difficult after the Vowel + [l] words are stabilized. When [l] + Vowel words are introduced, watch the tongue from a side view to be sure the back of the tongue is not elevating with the tip.

[l] + Vowel*

[li]

lea	plead	link	clink
lee	please	linger	clinic
leak	bleak	lit	clinch
league	bleed	litter	clip
leaguer	bleach	literal	cliff
legal	bleacher	literature	glitter
lead	flea	little	glint
leader	flee	lid	glisten
lean	fleet	linoleum	glimpse
lien	fleece	linen	slick
lease		lint	sling
least	xx	linseed	slink
leash		lilt	slit
leisure	ringleader	lily	slip
leech	gasoline	list	slipper
liege	vaseline	listen	slim
leap	asleep	lisp	sliver
leapfrog	oversleep	lizard	blink
leaf	replete	lip	bliss
leaflet	deplete	lipstick	blister
leave	complete	liberate	blizzard
leaves	displease	liberal	blimp
leeway	jubilee	liberty	flick
	sublease	limb	fling
x	nosebleed	limit	flit
	athlete	limp	flint
clear		limber	flip
clean		lift	flimsy
glee	[lɪ]	live	
gleam		livid	
sleek	leer		xx
sleet	lick		
sleep	licorice	x	yearling
sleeve	liquid		barley
plea	ligament	click	garlic
pleat	ling	cling	scarlet
			careless

*Most words ending with ed, s, and ing are not listed but should be considered if additional words are needed.

weakling
ticklish
eclipse
wreckless
necklace
crackling
chocolate
nuclear
inkling
anklet
Franklin
thankless
ugly*
singly
English
artless
courtly
gently
ghastly
giblet
goblet
goblin
medley
badly
oddly
hardly
kindling
enlist
only
bracelet
useless
cowslip
parsley
porcelain
grizzly
muslin

sapling
chaplain
poplin
discipline
couplet
explicit
simply
amply
accomplish
ably
tablet
establish
bobolink
public
assembly
numbly
afflict
inflict
conflict
lovely
earthling

[le]

lay
layer
lake
late
latex
laid
lady
ladybug
ladle
lain
lace
lazy
label

labor
lame
lathe

x

clay
claim
glaze
glacier
sleigh
slate
slain
play
plate
plain
place
blade
blaze
blame
flake
flame
flavor

xx

bouclé
acclaim
declaim
proclaim
exclaim
conclave
everglade
outlay
inlay

unlace
isolate
oscillate
translate
replay
replace
seaplane
triplane
airplane
interplay
fireplace
display
displace
explain
complain
complaint
contemplate
ablaze
deflate
deflation
aflame

[lɛ]

lecture
leg
leggings
legacy
let
letter
lets
lettuce
led
leaden
lent
lend

*Many words ending with ly are not listed but should be considered if more words are needed.

lens
less
lesson
lest
ledger
legend
leopard
leapt
lemon
left
leather

x

clench
clever
glare
glen
sled
slender
sledge
slept
plenty
pleasant
pleasure
pledge
blare
blend
bless
blemish
flare
fleck
fled
flesh

xx

eclair
declare
neglect

outlet
intellect
heedless
adolescent
unless
bobsled
triplex
duplex
perplex
replenish
capillary
aplenty
complex
complexion
sublet
reflex
reflect
deflect
inflection
athletic

[laɪ]

lie
liar
like
light
lighter
lightning
lied
line
lining
lion
lice
license
liable
library
librarian

lime
life
lifesaver
live
lilac

x

client
climb
climate
glide
sly
slight
slide
slice
slime
ply
pliers
blight
blind
fly
flyer
flight
flies

xx

starlight
hairline
recline
decline
incline
footlight
outline
headlight
sunlight
moonlight
enlighten

enliven
penalize
dislike
backslide
horselaugh
apply
reply
multiply
supply
comply
compliance
horseplay
oblige
sublime
butterfly
firefly
housefly
civilize

[læ]

lariat
lack
lax
lacquer
lag
lank
language
lad
ladder
lantern
land
landscape
landmark
lance
lass
lasso
last
lash

latch
lap
lapse
lamb
lamp
laminate
laugh
laughter
lava
lavender
lavish
lath
lather

x

clarinet
clang
clank
clatter
clad
clan
class
classic
clasp
clash
clap
clam
clamp
glad
glance
glass
slack
slang
slat
slant
slander
slash

slap
slab
slam
plank
platter
platform
plaid
plan
plant
planter
plaster
plastic
black
blacken
blank
blanket
bland
blast
flag
flank
flat
flatter
flannel
flask
flash
flashlight
flap

xx

backlash
outclass
hourglass
spyglass
sunglass
wineglass
Atlantic
outlandish
mainland

stepladder
replant
eggplant
transplant
explanatory
gangplank
avalanche
northland

[lɑ]

la
lark
lard
larder
large
larva
lock
lot
lotto
lollipop
lodge
logic
lob
lobby
lobster
llama

x

clock
clog
clot
closet
cloth
slot
slosh
slop
slobber

plot
plod
plop
blah
block
blot
blotter
blossom
phlox
flog
flop

xx

o'clock
conglomerate
deadlock
padlock
unlock
enlarge
dislodge
fuselage
camouflage

[lɔ]

law
lawyer
log
long
lawn
laundry
launch
loss
lost
loft

x

claw

93

clause
gloss
slaw
flaw
floss

xx

backlog
tablecloth
broadcloth
cheesecloth
outlaw
headlong
inlaw
applaud
applause
oblong

[lo]

low
lore
locate
location
local
load
loan
lone
lotion
lope
lobe
loam
loaf
loaves
lower

x

chlorin
chloroform

cloak
close
clothes
clove
clover
glow
glory
gloat
globe
slow
slogan
slope
blow
flow
floor
floral
florist
float
flown

xx

cyclone
foreclose
bedclothes
enclose
disclose
aglow
antelope
cantaloupe
dislocate
deplore
diploma
shipload
explore
explode
explosion
implore
overflow

buffalo
afloat

[lʊ]

lure
look
looking
looked
lookout

xx

outlook
onlooker
influence
influenza

[lu]

Lou
lukewarm
loot
lieutenant
loose
loosen
lose
loop
lubricate
loom
louver
Lutheran

x

clue
glue
gloom
slough
sloop

plume
blue
bloom
flew
flute
fluid

xx

heirloom
seclude
exclude
include
conclude
recluse
igloo

[lʌ]

luck
lux
luxury
lug
luggage
lung
London
lunch
luncheon
lunge
luster
lush
luscious
lump
lumber
love

x

cluck
clung

94

clutter
cluster
club
clumsy
clump
glut
glum
glove
slug
slung
slunk
slush
slum
slump
slumber
pluck
plug
plus
plum
plump
blood
blunt
blunder
blush
bluff
flung
flunk
flutter
flood
flush
fluff

xx

potluck
unlucky

surplus
influx

[lə]

lagoon
lapel
lament

xx

garland
declaration
exclamation
England
negligence
atlas
cutlass
bedlam
hoodlum
woodland
inland
Iceland
excellent
application
duplicate
diplomat
explanation
complicate
compliment
implement
amplify
simplify
obligate
sublimate
pablum
problem
emblem

semblance
conflagrate
southland

[lɚ]

xx

parlor
burglar
angler
rattler
butler
antler
counselor
stapler
poplar
sampler
cobbler
gobbler
muffler

[lɝ]

lurk
learn
learned
lurch

x

clerk
clergy
slur
slurp
blur
blurb

[l aʊ]

lout
loud
lounge
louse

x

cloud
clown
slouch
plow
blouse
flower

xx

snowplow
cauliflower
sunflower

[l ɔɪ]

loiter
Lloyd
loin
loyal

xx

disloyal
deploy
employ
employment
exploit

95

Vowel + [l]

[il]

eel
heal
heel
he'll
real
reel
creel
newsreel
keel
teal
genteel
steal
steel
deal
kneel
chenille
seal
conceal
zeal
she'll
peel
appeal
repeal
automobile
meal
feel
veal
reveal
wheel
cogwheel
we'll
squeal

xx

yield*

shield
field
outfield
infield
wield

wheelbarrow
fielder

[ɪl]

ill
hill
foothill
downhill
rill
grill
trill
drill
shrill
frill
thrill
kill
skill
gill
till
still
distill
reptile
dill
daffodil
nil
sill
chill
pill

spill
bill
mill
fill
refill
servile
vaudeville
anvil
will
quill
tranquil
twill

xx

silk
bilk
milk
hilt
tilt
stilt
jilt
built
wilt
quilt
guild
build
kiln
bilge
film
filth

billion
brilliant
civilian

billiard
familiar
milkman
milkweed
silkworm
pilgrim
kilter
guilty
filter
filtrate
killdeer
children
building
mildew
wilderness
bewilder
illness
hillside
millstone
millstream
killjoy
pillbox
billboard
Gilbert
filbert
skillful
billfold
silver

[el]

ale
ail
hale
hail

---

*Words ending with s and ed are not listed but if [lz] or additional [ld] blends are desired, these endings may be used with many of the final [l] words listed above. Most words ending with ing are not listed for the blends.

exhale
yale
rail
derail
trail
Braille
frail
kale
percale
scale
gale
regale
tale
tail
retail
detail
curtail
cattail
cottontail
fantail
stale
horsetail
bobtail
dovetail
dale
nail
fingernail
snail
hobnail
sale
sail
assail
mainsail
topsail
shale
jail
pail
pale
bale

bail
mail
male
female
fail
vale
veil
avail
travail
prevail
whale
wail
quail

xx

regalia
railroad
sailcloth
hailstorm
hailstone
salesroom
salesman
stalemate
paleface
baleful
railway

[ɛl]

ell
yell
tell
foretell
pastel
dell
knell
personnel
sell
cell

carousel
excel
shell
eggshell
nutshell
bombshell
gel
repel
propel
spell
expel
compel
bell
smell
fell
well
farewell
quell
inkwell
dwell
swell

xx

elk
dealt
knelt
pelt
belt
melt
smelt
felt
heartfelt
welt
held
weld
else
belch
squelch

help
yelp
kelp
elm
helm
realm
elf
self
myself
thyself
ourself
yourself
itself
oneself
shelf
delve
shelve
twelve
health
stealth
wealth

delta
shelter
swelter
elder
eldest
seldom
escelsior
felspar
helpful
shellproof
elbow
spellbound
bellboy
helmet
elfish
selfish

shellfish
belfry
welfare
velvet
healthy
wealthy

[aɪl]

I'll
isle
aisle
rile
trial
guile
tile
style
textile
dial
crocodile
senile
exile
reconcile
pile
compile
bile
mile
smile
file
profile
vile
while

xx

child
grandchild
mild
wild

wildcat
milestone
milepost

[æl]

corral
canal
shall
pal

xx

shalt
alp
scalp
valve
bivalve

stallion
dahlia
medallion
valiant
value
alcove
balcony
altitude
alto
contralto
calcium
algebra
nostalgia
alpaca
scalpel
album
albino
Balboa

alphabet
alphabetize
galvanize
salvia
salvage

[ɑl]

protocol
doll
menthol

xx

golf
solve
resolve
absolve
evolve
revolve
involve

soluble
voluble
volume
volcano
golfer
dolphin
insolvent

[ɔl]

all
awl
haul
hall
alcohol
overhaul
yawl
overall

crawl
trawl
sprawl
enthrall
call
recall
catcall
jackal
gall
tall
stall
install
bookstall
parasol
shawl
pall
appall
bawl
ball
snowball
football
handball
baseball
maul
mall
small
fall
befall
snowfall
pitfall
footfall
windfall
wall
squall

xx

halt
salt

assault
basalt
somersault
exalt
malt
fault
vault
scald
bald
false

already
ballroom
walrus
falcon
alter
altar
alternate
alteration
altogether
halter
Baltimore
Baltic
falter
alder
cauldron
walnut
also
gallstone
balsam
falsify
falsehood
palsy
smallpox
wallpaper
almighty
almost
almanac

hallmark
installment
always
stalwart
although

[ol]

oriole
hole
porthole
roll
role
parole
scroll
troll
control
stroll
droll
coal
charcoal
goal
toll
stole
extol
dole
condole
knoll
sole
soul
insole
console
poll
pole
bowl
mole
foal

colt
jolt
bolt
molt
volt
revolt
old
hold
cold
scold
gold
marigold
told
sold
bold
mold
fold

polka
polecat
poultice
poultry
molten
holdup
holder
potholder
colder
shoulder
boulder
smolder
folder
golden
goldenrod
goldfish
wholesale
wholesome
holster

coleslaw
soldier

[ʊl]

granule
full
jarful
basketful
bagful
handful
painful
spoonful
boxful
dishful
cupful
armful
brimful
pull
bull
wool

wolf
wolves

bulldog
bulldoze
pulpit
fullback
Pullman
pulmonary
bullfight
bullfinch
bullfrog
fulfill

[ul]

rule	hulk	emulsion	special
overrule	sulk	convulsion	social
cool	bulk	culture	agile
school	cult	agriculture	fragile
preschool	adult	vulture	angel
ghoul	insult	culprit	careful
tool	consult	sculptor	useful
tulle	exult	pulpwood	equal
stool	result	mulberry	
footstool	tumult	culminate	
duel	pulse	sulfur	xx
nodule	repulse	sulfuric	
pool	impulse	culvert	royalty
spool	convulse	pulverize	realty
cesspool	gulch		specialty
fool	mulch	[əl]	

xx

peculiar
schoolyard
schoolhouse
schoolroom
schoolgirl
schoolteacher
schoolmate
foolscap

[ʌl]

hull	bulge	ideal	earl
	gulp	material	hurl
	pulp	remedial	curl
	bulb	trial	girl
	gulf	continual	pearl
	engulf	visual	purl
		actual	burl
	skullcap	gradual	furl
	bulky	individual	whirl
	vulgar	cruel	twirl
	ulterior	fuel	swirl
	ultimatum	squirrel	
	cultivate	royal	xx
	multiple	spaniel	
	multitude	barrel	world
hull	ultra	oral	
cull	sultry	quarrel	[aʊl]
skull	ulcer	mural	
gull	pulsate	general	howl
dull	emulsify	natural	yowl
null	expulsion	several	growl
mull	compulsion	central	trowel

[ʒl]

[ɜl]

	[ɔɪl]		xx
prowl	oil	topsoil	oilcloth
scowl	broil	subsoil	oilskin
towel	coil	spoil	[jul]
jowl	recoil	boil	you'll
foul	gargoyle	parboil	yule
fowl	toil	foil	ridicule
vowel	soil	voile	mule

Vowel + [l] + Vowel (The vowel following [l] is noted.)

[li]

elite
delete
release
relief
relieve
colleague
obsolete
police
policeman
valise
belief
believe
alleviate

[lɪ]

chameleon
helium
heartily
readily
speedily
bodily
silly
chilly
Billy
filly
heavily
delirious
illiterate
skillet
belittle
humiliate
affiliate
penicillin
penniless
religion
village
deliver
daily
grayling

alien
alias
jelly
dwelling
helicopter
pelican
pellet
Helen
cellist
relish
intelligible
filing
eyelet
alley
rally
galley
tally
valley
ballyhoo
metallic
palate
mallet
pallid
valid
challenge
palace
malice
holly
trolley
collie
dolly
Polly
folly
volley
finale
tamale
frolic
colic

wallet
polish
abolish
demolish
college
olive
polliwog
calling
holy
olio
polio
folio
rolling
bowling
foliage
petroleum
pulley
bully
pullet
bullet
truly
coolie
duly
foolish
julep
gully
broccoli
generally
family
violet
violin
masculine
insulin
solicit
realism
collision
overly
early
surly

burly
curlicue
doily

[le]

relay
delay
elate
relate
elation
relation
chalet
ballet
articulate
calculate
circulate
regulate
coagulate
granulate
stipulate
manipulate
populate
cumulate
simulate
formulate
allay
Chevrolet
correlate
percolate
insulate
congratulate

[lɛ]

elect
electric
electron
relent
eleven

silex
bolero
collect
parallel
convalescent
allege
celebrity

[laɪ]

beeline
feline
rely
delight
daylight
twilight
towline
July
alike
aline
polite
allied
collide
align
alliance
centralize
generalize
sterilize
paralyze
alive
saliva

[læ]

relax
elastic
elapse
relapse
elaborate

eyelash
shellac
wonderland
alas
molasses
collapse
collaborate
overland
overlap
burlap

[lɑ]

illogical
alarm
allot
ocelot
echelon
velocity
galoshes
chronologic
jalopy

[lɔ]

elongate
hayloft
bylaw
prologue
dialogue
along
prolong
belong
aloft
waterlog
forlorn
furlong

[lo]

pillow

billow
willow
elope
halo
hello
yellow
cello
bellow
fellow
silo
hallow
Halloween
callow
tallow
sallow
shallow
fallow
hollow
follow
wallow
swallow
solo
polo
aloha
piccolo
bungalow
below
galore
alone
baloney
abalone
colonial
envelope

[lʊ]

allure
overlook

[lu]

prelude
elude
delude
elusive
illusion
delusion
illuminate
aluminum
hullabaloo
alleluia
salute
absolute
pollute
allude
balloon
hallucination
solution
revolution
allusion
collusion
aloof

[lʌ]

illustrious
beloved
Columbia

[lə]

gorilla
mantilla
vanilla
chinchilla
artillery
filigree
futility
facility
agility

103

ability	highland	quality	miller
stability	silence	holiday	pillar
humility	calla	pollen	caterpillar
military	calorie	colony	sailor
villain	gallery	Holland	cellar
millinery	salary	volunteer	pallor
illustrate	galaxy	policy	valor
syllable	allocate	geology	mallard
filibuster	calico	biology	allergy
filament	ballad	apologize	collar
kilowatt	malady	scallop	scholar
gala	gallon	solemn	dollar
available	gallant	column	squalor
celery	talent	columbine	collarbone
eloquent	valentine	alamode	solar
delicate	calendar	qualify	polar
elegant	balance	kola	molar
telegram	callus	viola	fuller
delegate	Dallas	colon	cruller
skeleton	ballast	stolen	color
gelatin	fallacy	swollen	circular
fidelity	gallop	Poland	curricular
relative	caliber	bulletin	jocular
felon	alibi	tulip	binocular
repellant	Alabama	gullible	particular
telescope	alabaster	nullify	muscular
jealous	halibut	formula	regular
elegy	fallible	fraudulent	jugular
intelligent	alum	ambulance	singular
celebrate	Alamo	ridiculous	angular
element	alimony	nebulous	rectangular
elephant	salamander	fabulous	granular
telephone	gallivant	cumulous	popular
cellophane	Colorado	curriculum	consular
elevator	holocaust	gondola	chancellor
relevant	molecule	peninsula	[1ɚ]
television	solitary	spatula	alert
pilot	politics	Pamela	allergic

[laʊ]

allow
allowance
aloud

[lɔɪ]

alloy
celluloid
sirloin
purloin

[lju]

deluge

Final and Medial [l] Blends*

[rl]

Carl
gnarl
snarl

[kl]

trickle
prickle
numerical
tickle
article
particle
practical
cuticle
nickel
icicle
tricycle
bicycle
pickle
heckle
freckle
speckle
motorcycle
tackle
shackle
cockle
bifocal
vocal
honeysuckle
chuckle
buckle
spectacle
barnacle
miracle

circle
sparkle
crinkle
sprinkle
periwinkle
ankle
rankle
uncle

xx

faculty
huckleberry

[gl]

eagle
regal
giggle
jiggle
wiggle
finagle
inveigle
haggle
straggle
waggle
goggle
joggle
ogle
frugal
bugle
struggle
snuggle
juggle
smuggle
gurgle

gargle
tingle
single
shingle
mingle
angle
triangle
strangle
tangle
rectangle
dangle
jangle
spangle
mangle
fangle
jungle
bungle

xx

angleworm

[tl]

beetle
it'll
brittle
hospital
whittle
natal
fatal
kettle
nettle
settle
petal

metal
title
entitle
recital
vital
rattle
prattle
cattle
tattle
chattel
battle
bottle
total
brutal
futile
scuttle
subtle
shuttle
capital
turtle
fertile
startle
chortle
mortal
portal
oriental
parental
continental
gentle
mental
instrumental
fundamental
ornamental
mantle

*Plurals are not included, so if triple blends ending in [lz] are desired, an s may be added to many of the final blends above. If triple blends ending in [ld] are desired, add ed to many of the final blends above.

dismantle
horizontal
crystal
pedestal
pistol

xx

rattletrap
rattlesnake
battleship
shuttlecock

[dl]

needle
riddle
griddle
middle
fiddle
cradle
treadle
medal
peddle
idle
bridal
addle
saddle
paddle
coddle
model
waddle
dawdle
yodel
doodle
noodle
feudal
cuddle
puddle
fuddle

hurdle
kindle
spindle
dwindle
handle
candle
scandal
sandal
fondle
bundle

xx

fiddletsticks
middleman
middleweight
meddlesome
saddlebag
candlestick

[nl]

penal
marginal
spinal
final
channel
gunnel
tunnel
funnel
sentinel
conditional
sensational
sectional
exceptional
conventional
rational
national
occasional
original
criminal

nominal
juvenile
kernel
colonel
eternal
internal
paternal
maternal
journal
infernal
signal
personal

xx

penalty

[sl]

bristle
epistle
missal
thistle
whistle
basal
wrestle
trestle
nestle
vessel
tassel
docile
fossil
hustle
rustle
tussle
bustle
muscle
mussel
corpuscle

domicile
reversal
parcel
dorsal
morsel
axle
pretzel
stencil
pencil
cancel
consul
tonsil
council
counsel
capsule

[zl]

easel
drizzle
frizzle
sizzle
chisel
fizzle
nasal
embezzle
frazzle
dazzle
nozzle
accusal
refusal
guzzle
puzzle
damsel

xx

measles
hazelnut

[pl]

steeple
people
ripple
cripple
triple
participle
staple
maple
apple
grapple
dapple
chapel
opal
scruple
principal
principle
Episcopal
municipal
couple
purple
gospel
simple
pimple
temple
ample
sample

xx

steeplechase
applesauce
applejack

[bl]

feeble
dribble
scribble
nibble
impossible
able
cable

gable
enable
table
stable
sable
fable
rebel
treble
pebble
dabble
hobble
cobble
gobble
wobble
squabble
noble
mobile
ruble
rubble
trouble
stubble
double
bubble
terrible
excitable
portable
convertible
edible
responsible
possible
excusable
sociable
capable
movable
garble
warble
nimble
symbol

thimble
tremble
assemble
amble
ramble
scramble
bramble
gamble
shamble
humble
rumble
grumble
jumble
fumble

xx

troublesome
cobblestone
tablespoon
nobleman
bumblebee

[ml]

camel
enamel
mammal
caramel
normal
formal
dismal

[fl]

sniffle
rifle
trifle
stifle
raffle
baffle
awful
waffle

scuffle
shuffle

xx

scaffold
rifleman

[vl]

evil
medieval
weevil
drivel
snivel
civil
naval
devil
daredevil
rival
revival
survival
ravel
gravel
travel
gavel
grovel
novel
oval
hovel
shovel
festival
carnival
interval

xx

rivalry
cavalry
cavalcade
novelty
devilfish

r

[r]

[r]

Construction of the [r] *Word Lists*

1. There are five categories:
   a. the [r] followed by a vowel including initial [r] and initial and medial [r] blends [kr, skr, gr, tr, dr, ʃr, pr, spr, br, fr, θr] in that order.
   b. initial, medial, and final [ɚ] or [ɝ].
   c. the [r] preceded by a vowel including final [r] and final and medial [r] blends.
   d. the [r] preceded and followed by a vowel.
   e. words which may be difficult at the beginning of therapy.

2. The first words listed in the [r] + Vowel category require limited lip movement in production. Words requiring more lip movement are listed next.

3. Where appropriate, the [r] is combined with other consonants in the order which follows:
   [h, j, r, k, g, ŋ, t, d, n, l, s, z, ʃ, ʒ, tʃ, dʒ, p, b, m, f, v, θ, ð, hw, w].
   The words rack, rag, rang, rat, ran; or hair, care, tare, and dare illustrate some of these combinations. If a slight shift in vowels is desired, words such as reek, rake, wreck, rack, rock, and rook are found near the beginning of each list because [k] is combined with [r] after [h] and [j].

4. Where appropriate, the [r] is combined with vowels and diphthongs in the following order:
   [i, ɪ, e, ɛ, aɪ, æ, ɑ, ɔ, o, ʊ, u, ʌ, ə, ɚ, ɜ, ɝ, aʊ, ɔɪ, ju].

5. To facilitate the location of words in a category, initial [r] blends are noted by x, medial [r, ɚ, ɝ] by xx, and final [ɚ] by xxx.

Characteristics and Use of the [r] *Word Lists*

1. Choose words which are appropriate for the age and interests of the client. Many words are listed for high school students and adults but they would not be considered for small children. The lists also reflect

109

the relative frequency of each vowel in combination with [r]. For example, there are many more words beginning with [rɪ] than [rɔɪ].

2. Determine which sound combination is the easiest.
    a. If it is [ɝ], begin on pages 121–126.
    b. If it is [ɑr], begin on pages 128–129.
    c. If it is [r] + Vowel, begin on pages 113–120. Choose the vowel which makes the [r] production easiest. This frequently is [ɑ] or [ɔ].
    d. If it is a blend, begin with that blend on pages 113–120. Many children with inconsistent misarticulation of the [r] sound correctly articulate some initial [r] blends. Stabilize them.

3. It may or may not be desirable to proceed down the [r] + Vowel lists. If it is not desirable, it is a simple matter to skip to the next list. The first words listed require limited lip movement and are useful for clients who substitute [w] for [r].

4. The initial [r] blends are listed according to the vowel which follows them because the vowel influences the production of the blend. However, if a number of [gr] blends are desired, for example, they are easily found because the [gr] blends follow the [kr] and [skr] blends in each list.

Methods of Correcting the [r] Sound

The position of the tongue tip does not appear to be an important factor in the production of the [r] sound. The tip may be up, down, or in between depending upon the anatomical construction of the oral cavity. Of prime importance is the contact of the lateral borders of the tongue and the posterior molars or their gum ridge. The extreme posterior portion of the tongue must not be elevated or a nasal [r] will result.

Most speech specialists teach the [ɝ] rather than the [r] in the early stages of therapy. The auditory-visual method of teaching the [ɝ] is, of course, preferred. However, in some cases, the client is unable to say [ɝ] without additional assistance. The placement ideas which follow have been helpful in these instances. As will be pointed out, not all suggestions are accurate from an anatomic point of view but, if the problem is functional, they are practical and usually produce the desired results—an acceptable [ɝ] sound.

1.	Ask the child to imitate a fire siren [ɝ〰〰], a rooster crowing [ɝ-ɝ-ɝ-ɝ-ɝ], or a bear growling [ɡɝ]. Sometimes the suggestion, "Be sure your tongue is way up and way back," is all that is necessary to help him find the proper tongue placement. If further help is needed, place your hand, palm down, on the top of the child's head and say, "Try to touch my hand with your tongue as you say [ɝ]." Obviously this is impossible but many children get the idea of elevating the lateral borders of the tongue by this suggestion.

2.	Ask the client to say [i]. Call attention to the contact of the gum ridge and the lateral borders of the tongue. Ask the client to increase the tongue pressure to really feel the contact. Ask the client to pull the tip of the tongue back without breaking the lateral contact to say [ɝ]. The [i] is particularly good because the lips are pulled back and tend to discourage the [ʊ] which is frequently substituted for the [ɝ]. However, the [n, d, t, ʒ, ʃ] may be used in the same manner as the [i] and are easier for some clients. Tongue action may be illustrated by cupping the hands together and drawing back the finger tips of the hand which is on the bottom.

3.	Ask the client to say [ɑr]. Demonstrate to the client the way the tongue should be raised by extending your right hand, palm down (representing the tongue in the [ɑ] position). Raise the knuckles (the large joints which join the fingers to the hand) and extend the fingers slightly downward (representing the [r] position). Make an arch with the thumb and forefinger of your left hand pointing downward to represent the roof of the mouth and the alveolar ridges where lateral tongue contact is to be made. Retaining the arch, place the thumb of your left hand on the side of the raised knuckle of the forefinger of your right hand and place the tip of the forefinger of your left hand on the side of the raised knuckle of the little finger of your right hand. Demonstrate the movement by extending your right hand to the [ɑ] position and raising the knuckles to touch the thumb and forefinger of your left hand. Ask the client to say [ɑr] as you demonstrate.

4.	With a tongue depressor, stroke the lateral borders of the tongue and the posterior gum ridges. Ask the client to make contact between the stroked areas and say [ɝ].

5.	Place your thumb and forefinger on the client's cheeks and push against the upper posterior molars. Ask the client to push against your fingers with the sides of his tongue as he says [ɝ]. Here again, the instructions are not strictly accurate but give the idea of tongue placement to some clients.

6.   Some speech specialists teach initial $[r]$ + Vowel through the $[ɜ]$ as $[ɜr]$ + Vowel. For example, ask the child to be a fire siren $[ɜ \sim\sim\sim\sim]$ and add ed for the word *red*. Prolong the $[ɜ]$ and do not pause before the ed. The same results may be obtained by blending a word ending with $[ɚ]$ with a word beginning with $[r]$ such as *her red* or *mother ran*. The $[ɚ]$ will be **prolonged** and the ed or the an added without pausing or inserting another sound. The first of these two techniques is not strictly correct phonetically speaking because $[ɜrʌn]$ is not the correct pronunciation of *run*. However, experience shows that most children drop the $[ɜ]$ very quickly when the words are put into sentences. If this does not occur naturally, the suggestion, "Say the first part of the word faster" is usually all that is necessary.

7.   If the $[w]$ is substituted for the initial $[r]$, the first words listed in the $[r]$ + Vowel section are particularly useful because they require limited lip movement. If the client reverts to the $[w]$ substitution, use a mirror to call attention to the puckered lips, ask the client to smile in an exaggerated manner, or inhibit the movement by pushing the upper lip back against the upper teeth with your thumb and forefinger.

112

[r] + Vowel*

[ri]

reek	greedy	increase	relax
recall	green	concrete	relate
regal	grease	discreet	relent
retail	grief	ice cream	release
read	tree	agree	risk
reed	trio	degree	wrist
real	treat	disagree	recite
reel	treason	agreeable	receipt
really	streak	ingredient	recede
relay	street	gangrene	recess
realize	stream	entreat	resign
reason	streamline	mistreat	result
wreath	dream	extreme	resist
wreathe	shriek	daydream	
	preheat	appreciate	request
reach	preen	depreciate	renew
region	precede	supreme	religion
reject	preschool	debris	relation
reap	priest	abbreviate	reliable
ream	preach	abbreviation	relief
remodel	prefix	antifreeze	relieve
reef	spree		receive
	breed	### [rɪ]	respect
x	breeze		respond
	breech	rig	response
creak	breach	regain	resolve
creek	free	ring	rich
creed	freak	rink	ridge
creel	frequent	wrinkle	reject
crease	freedom	written	rigid
creep	freeze	retain	rejoice
cream	three	rid	rip
screen	threesome	ridden	ripple
screech		riddle	reply
scream	xx	ridiculous	repeat
greet		rinse	rib
greed	decree	rely	

*Words ending with s, ed, and ing are not listed

ribbon
rim
remit
remote
remedial
remain
remiss
remove
rift
refuse
rivet
revoke
revenge
revolt
rhythm

x

cricket
critic
criticize
creative
cringe
christen
crystal
crisp
Christmas
crib
cribbage
crimson
script
scribble
scrimmage
grit
grid
griddle
grin
grill
gristle

grizzly
grip
grim
trick
trickle
trinket
trill
trip
triple
tribute
trim
strict
string
strip
drink
drill
drizzle
drip
drift
shrink
shrill
shrimp
shrivel
prickle
pretty
pretend
predict
print
prince
princess
principal
principle
precise
prim
primitive
prevent
privilege
sprig

spring
sprinkle
sprint
brick
bring
brink
brittle
brisk
bridge
friction
fringe
frill
frisk
frigid
thrill
thrift
thrifty

xx

hickory
secret
sacred
discriminate
description
subscription
tigress
chagrin
angry
congregate
pilgrim
psychiatry
metric
patriot
patriotic
hatred
putrid
mattress
nutrition

victory
actress
doctrine
entry
country
pantry
wintry
contribute
poultry
history
industry
pastry
tapestry
industrial
industrious
gastric
district
constrict
bowstring
ostrich
padre
laundry
sundry
adrift
enrich
cavalry
chivalry
glycerin
misery
slippery
apprehend
apricot
blueprint
footprint
culprit
desperate
lubricate
abridge
infringe

belfry
every
everyday
everything
everybody
everyone
maverick
average
favorite

[re]

ray
rake
rate
raid
radiate
radius
rain
reign
rayon
rail
race
raise
raisin

radio
radium
rainbow
range
railway
ratio
ration
rage
rabies
rave
raven

x

crate

cradle
crane
crayon
crepe
crayfish
crave
scrape
grey
grate
great
grade
grain
grace
grape
graham
grave
gravy
tray
trait
trade
train
trail
trace
stray
straight
strain
strange
drake
drain
drape
pray
prey
praise
spray
sprain
bray
brake
break

braid
brain
Braille
brace
bracelet
brave
freight
frail
phrase
frame

xx

integrate
migrate
degrade
downgrade
ingrain
disgrace
disgraceful
integration
penetrate
citrate
outrage
astray
eyestrain
illustrate
demonstrate
illustration
hydrate
enrage
appraise
hombre
celebrate
vibrate
membrane
embrace
celebration
afraid

wreck
recognize
rectangle
retina
red
ready
readily
wren
rent
rend
rest
wrestle

wrench
relative
relish
rescue
recipe
recitation
resolution
repetition
reputation
reptile
rebel
remedy

x

crest
crept
credit
credible
trek
tread
trend
trench
trestle
tremble

115

strength
strenuous
stress
stretch
dread
drench
dress
dredge
shred
pretzel
press
present
precious
spread
breakfast
bred
bread
breadth
breath
freckle
fret
friend
frenzy
French
fresh
threat
thread
thresh

xx

decrepit
aggressive
digress
address
undress
already
depress
suppress

impress
express
bedspread
impressive
depression
impression
expression
inbred
umbrella
befriend

[raɪ]

rye
rite
right
write
riot
ride
rind
rice
rise

rhino
rhinestone
ripe
ripen
rhyme
rifle
rival

x

cry
cried
crisis
cries
crime
scribe
grind

gripe
grime
try
trite
tried
triad
triangle
trial
trice
tricycle
tries
tribe
trifle
strike
stride
stripe
strife
strive
dry
dried
dries
drive
driveway
pry
pride
pried
price
pries
prize
prime
private
spry
sprite
bright
brighten
bride
bridle
brine

bribe
fry
fright
frighten
fried
Friday
fries
thrice
thrive

xx

describe
subscribe
contrive
handwriting
downright
sunrise
alright
upright
surprise
deprive

[ræ]

rack
racket
rag
rang
rank
rat
rattle
rattlesnake
ran
rant
rancid
rally
wrath

racoon
radish

random
ransom
ranch
rash
ration
rational
wrap
rap
rapt
rapid
rabbit
rabble
ram
ramp
rampage
ramble
raft
raffle

x

crack
crank
crash
crab
cram
cramp
craft
scratch
scrap
scramble
gratitude
grant
grand
grass
grasp
graduate
gradual
grab
gram

graph
gravity
gravel
track
transit
trash
tragic
trap
traffic
travel
straddle
strand
strap
drag
dragon
drank
drab
draft
shrank
practice
prank
prance
sprang
brag
brad
bran
brand
branch
brass
fraction
frank
thrash

xx

bookrack
democrat
handicraft
woodcraft

bluegrass
congratulate
diagram
telegram
photograph
telegraph
mimeograph
attract
detract
contract
subtract
diaphragm

[rɑ]

rah
rock
rocket
rot
rotten
rod
Ron
rosin

rob
robin
romp

x

crock
crocodile
chronic
chronicle
crop
groggy
grotto
trot
trod
trolley

tropic
trombone
drop
drama
prod
product
pronto
process
prop
probable
problem
promise
prompt
profit
broccoli
bronco
bronze
frock
frog
frolic
throttle
throb

xx

electron
dogtrot
bedrock
dewdrop
gumdrop
melodrama
approximate
shamrock

[rɔ]

raw
wrong
rawhide

x

craw
crawl

117

cross
scrawl
straw
strong
draw
drawn
drawl
prawn
sprawl
brought
broad
broadcast
broth
fraud
frost
frosty
frostbite
froth
throng

xx

across
hydraulic
abroad
defrost

[ro]

row
rogue
rote
wrote
rotate
road
rode
rodeo
rodent
role
roll

roast
rose
rosy
roach
rope
robe
robot
rowboat
robust
roam
Rome
romaine
romance

x

crow
croak
crocus
chrome
scroll
grow
groan
gross
grove
troll
stroke
stroll
drone
droll
drove
protein
protest
prone
pronoun
prose
probe
broke
broach
froze

throw
throat
throne

xx

microbe
escrow
Negro
engross
control
patrol
petroleum
atrocious
electrode
sunstroke
enroll
approach
unbroken
bathrobe

[ru]

rook
rookie

x

crook
brook

xx

congruity
quadruple

[ru]

rue
root
routine
rutabaga

rude
ruin
rule
roulette
roost
rouge
ruby
room
roommate
roof
ruthless

x

crew
crude
croon
cruel
cruise
croup
screw
grew
group
groom
groove
true
truly
truce
troop
truth
strew
drew
drool
droop
shrew
shrewd
prude
prune
proof

118

prove
spruce
brew
brute
brutal
brood
brunette
bruin
bruise
broom
fruit
fruitcake
threw

xx

ecru
checkroom
cloakroom
intrude
intrusion
Andrew
bedroom
ballroom
classroom
lunchroom
approve
disapprove
improve

[rʌ]

rug
rugged
rung
rut
ruddy
run
runt
rusk
rust

rusty
rustle

rush
Russia
rub
rubble
rubbish
rum
rumpus
rumple
rumble
rumba
rough
roughen
ruffian
ruffle

x

crunch
crust
crush
crutch
crumb
crumple
crumble
scrub
scrubby
grunt
grudge
grub
grumble
gruff
truck
trunk
trust
trudge
trouble
troublesome

trump
trumpet
struck
struggle
strung
strut
strum
drug
druggist
drunk
drudge
drum
drumstick
shrug
shrunk
shrub
sprung
brunt
brush
front
from
thrust
thrush

xx

bankrupt
begrudge
entrust
destruction
distrust
obstruct
construct
construction
humdrum
abrupt
affront

[rə]

ravine

x

cravat
strategic
dramatic
pronounce
propose
provide

xx

okra
acrobat
sacrifice
microphone
microscope
mediocrity
integrity
emigrant
bibliography
congress
mongrel
citron
patron
matron
neutral
citrus
nitrogen
metropolitan
detriment
petrify
intricate
introduce
contradict
contribution
entrance
central
centralize
extra
nostril
apostrophe

119

catastrophe
hydrant
hydroplane
cathedral
hundred
hindrance
cauldron
children
miserable
apron
April
apropos
cypress
cobra
algebra
zebra
numeral
numerous

difference
indifference
Chevrolet
anthropology

[rau]

row
rout
round
rouse

x

kraut
crowd
crown
crouch

ground
growl
grouse
grouch
trout
trounce
trowel
drought
drown
drowsy
shroud
proud
prowl
sprout
brow
brown
browse
frown

aground
background

[rɔɪ]

Roy
royal
royalty

x

broil

xx

destroy
adroit
embroil

[ɝ] and [ɜ]

err
irk
urn
earn
earnest
earl
early
erst
urchin
urge
herb
urban
urbane
ermine
earth
earthen
earthquake

[h-]

her
hurt
hurtle
heard
herd
hurdle
hernia
hurl
hearse
herself
hers
hermit

[k-]

cur
curt
curtain
courtesy
curd

curdle
kernel
curl
curlicue
curse
cursive
kerchief
curb
curfew
curve

xxx

beaker
knicker
slicker
flicker
bicker
vicar
wicker
acre
taker
shaker
baker
homemaker
checker
woodpecker
lacquer
cocker
talker
walker
ocher
mediocre
lucre
tucker
pucker
occur
massacre
incur

tinker
anchor
canker
tanker
conquer
whisker

xx

skirt
scourge

skirmish
scurvy
excursion
neckerchief
handkerchief

[g-]

gurgle
gird
girl
girth

xxx

eager
leaguer
meager
digger
vinegar
jigger
bigger
vigor
beggar
tiger
stagger
dagger
swagger

logger
ogre
sugar
cougar
linger
finger
anger
longer
hunger
vulgar

xx

haggard

fingernail

[t-]

turkey
turquoise
turtle
turn
turnip
tournament
terse
turpentine
term
terminal
termite
turmoil
turf

xxx

teeter
liter
cheater
Peter
skitter

121

deter
litter
glitter
flitter
bitter
cater
educator
commentator
waiter
equator
letter
setter
better
lighter
miter
hatter
scatter
latter
clatter
platter
flatter
chatter
spatter
batter
matter
fatter
otter
totter
blotter
daughter
slaughter
water
motor
tutor
suitor
utter
cutter
gutter
stutter

clutter
shutter
putter
sputter
butter
mutter
janitor
monitor
diameter
goiter
loiter
pewter
victor
nectar
collector
actor
benefactor
doctor
splinter
winter
enter
center
canter
banter
saunter
hunter
counter
kilter
filter
shelter
alter
altar
halter
falter
canister
banister
sinister
minister
blister

sister
mister
waster
pester
fester
aster
caster
plaster
disaster
pastor
master
faster
impostor
foster
luster
cluster
bluster
fluster
muster
gangster
monster
holster
bolster
lobster
captor
chapter
after
laughter

xx

jitters
intern
lantern
stern
astern
eastern
western
custard
mustard

disturb
eternal

detergent
determine
jitterbug
bittersweet
watermelon
motorcycle
buttercup
butternut
butterscotch
buttermilk
butterfly
attorney
paternal
maternal
nocturnal
internal
intercede
yesterday
external
sturdy
sturgeon
stirrup

[d—]

dirt
dirty
derby
dearth

xxx

leader
cedar
consider
cider
spider

122

		xx	xx
ladder	holder	monarch	alert
madder	shoulder	inert	blurt
dodder	smolder		
fodder	boulder	inertia	allergic
odor		energy	colorful
shudder	**xx**	enervate	
powder	modern	monarchy	[s−]
gunpowder	standard		
hinder		[l−]	sir
tinder	modernize		circuit
cinder	tenderloin	lurk	circus
tender	tenderfoot	learn	circle
slender	wonderland	learned	certain
vendor	wilderness	lurch	certify
candor			surly
gander	[n−]	**xxx**	search
bystander	nurse		surge
slander	nerve	slur	surgeon
commander		blur	surplus
meander	**xxx**	pillar	surf
ponder		miller	surface
wander	inner	tailor	serve
squander	dinner	sailor	survey
launder	sinner	cellar	service
under	tenor	scholar	
plunder	liner	molar	**xxx**
blunder	miner	fuller	
thunder	minor	color	saucer
wonder	banner	singular	officer
calendar	manner	popular	boxer
lavender	manor	wiggler	answer
flounder	honor	angler	cancer
founder	donor	whistler	sponsor
bewilder	schooner	stapler	
elder	lunar	poplar	**xx**
wilder	gunner	gobbler	
alder	milliner	tumbler	assert
older	governor	muffler	insert
	joiner		conserve

assertion	[tʃ—]	germane	persuade
assertion	churr	germane	persuade
ascertain	churn	germicide	perch
insertion	churl		purchase
censorship	church	xxx	purge
	chirp		purpose
[z—]		voyager	purple
xxx	xxx	major	permit
		wager	permission
kaiser	teacher	ledger	perfect
geyser	pitcher	badger	perfume
incisor	nature	injure	
miser	catcher	ginger	xxx
	butcher	danger	
xx	signature	manger	housekeeper
	future	messenger	bookkeeper
scissors	picture	passenger	cheaper
observe	lecture	soldier	kipper
	manufacture		skipper
[ʃ—]	juncture	xx	dipper
	puncture		zipper
shirr	pincher	adjourn	chipper
shirk	venture		caper
shirt	vulture	gingersnap	taper
Shirley	gesture		paper
sherbert	pasture	[p—]	vapor
	posture		leper
xxx	moisture	purr	pepper
	mixture	perhaps	capper
kingfisher	capture	perk	hopper
washer		pert	copper
kosher	[dʒ—]	pertain	stopper
censure		purl	shopper
	jerk	pearl	pauper
[ʒ—]	jerkin	purse	super
xxx	journey	person	upper
	journal	personal	supper
leisure	journalism	personality	diaper
seizure	germ	persist	juniper
	German	percent	whisper
		pursue	

124

whimper
temper
hamper
damper
pamper

xx

spurt
expert
superb
leopard

impersonate
imperfect
jeopardize
supervise

[b−]

burr
berg
bird
burden
burn
burnt
burl
burlap
burst
birch
berth
birth

xxx

neighbor
labor
fiber
jabber
sober

caliber
timber
December
member
number
slumber

xx

bluebird
sunburn
suburb

liberty
gabardine
cumbersome

[m−]

myrrh
murky
mercy
merchant
merge
mirth

xxx

glimmer
slimmer
shimmer
hammer
stammer
clamor
glamour
bomber
homer
comber
tumor
consumer

hummer
summer
humor

xx

smirk
commerce
smirch
emerge
submerge

commercial
somersault

[f−]

fur
fir
forget
forgive
fertile
fern
furnace
furnish
first
forbid
firm
ferment

xxx

defer
differ
wafer
offer
gopher

chauffeur
suffer
sulphur
infer
confer

xx

effort
affirm
confirm
infirm

infirmity
infernal
affirmative

[v−]

vertical
verse
verge
verb
vermin

xxx

fever
liver
deliver
sliver
flavor
saver
favor
ever
never
lever
sever
diver
over

125

cover
discover
silver

xx

cavern
govern
adverb

overcast
overcoat
everglade
advertise
government

[hw—]

whirl
whirlpool

[w—]

were
work
word
weren't
world
worse
worst
worm
worth

xxx

network

handwork
housework
homework
squirt
awkward
catchwork
squirrel
twirl
swirl
squirm
bookworm
cutworm

[θ—]

Thursday
thermos
thermostat

xxx

ether
author
panther

[ð—]
xxx

either
neither
hither
dither
slither
wither

thither
heather
tether
leather
feather
pinfeather
whether
weather
gather
lather
father
other
mother
smother

[i—]
xxx

skier

[ɪ—]
xxx

nuclear
meteor

[e—]
xxx

layer
player
mayor

[aɪ—]
xxx

slyer

flyer
amplifier

[o—]
xxx

goer
lower

[aʊ—]
xxx

cower
tower
watchtower
dower
glower
flour
flower
Mayflower
sunflower
cauliflower
shower
power
empower
bower

[ɔɪ—]
xxx

employer
foyer

Vowel + [r] *

[ɪr]

ear	smear	stair	beware
here	cashmere	dare	square
hear	fear	ne'er	
year	sphere	millionaire	xx
gear	atmosphere	snare	
tear	veer	lair	scarce
volunteer	severe	eclair	downstairs
steer	queer	declare	bareheaded
austere		glair	warehouse
dear	xx	glare	haircut
deer		blare	heirloom
near	beard	flair	hairline
domineer	weird	flare	careless
pioneer	yearly	share	bearskin
mountaineer	nearly	chair	airplane
veneer	fierce	pair	bareback
souvenir	earshot	pare	chairman
leer	earphone	pear	careful
gondolier	cheerful	spare	barefoot
cavalier	earwig	despair	farewell
clear		impair	
sear	## [ɛr]	compare	## [ɑɪr]
sincere		bare	
sheer	air	bear	ire
shear	ere	mare	hire
cashier	heir	nightmare	tire
cheer	hare	fare	attire
jeer	hair	fair	entire
pier	mohair	affair	dire
peer	care	there	lyre
appear	scare	their	sire
disappear	tare	where	aspire
spear	tear	anywhere	conspire
bier	solitaire	ware	empire
beer	stare	wear	umpire
			vampire

*Most words ending with s and ed are not listed but should be considered if additional blends are desired. Most words ending with ing are not listed for the final blends.

mire
admire
fire
afire
sapphire
backfire
bonfire
gunfire
campfire
wire
choir
acquire
squire

xx

entirely
fireside
fireplace
fireman
firefly

[ɑr]

are
car
scar
cigar
tar
guitar
star
seminar
bizarre
char
jar
ajar
par
spar
bar

mar
far
afar
caviar
jaguar
boudoir
memoir

xx

arc
ark
hark
stark
dark
lark
shark
park
spark
bark
embark
mark
bookmark
postmark
Denmark
harken
darken
sparkle
arcade
architect
carcass
darkness
sarcasm
charcoal
parka
market

gargle
argue
cargo

bargain
embargo

art
heart
cart
tart
start
dart
chart
part
apart
depart
carton
startle
arty
Artic
artist
article
artesian
artificial
cartoon
party
partly
particle
apartment
department

hard
yard
card
discard
guard
lard
chard
bard
boulevard
harden
garden

pardon
ardent
hardy
hardly
yardstick
cardiac
guardian
gardenia
guardhouse
sardine

yarn
darn
barn
aren't
harness
carnation
carnival
garnet
garnish
tarnish
varnish
barnacle

Carl
gnarl
snarl
scarlet
garlic
garland
starlight
darling

sparse
farce
arson
parcel
parsnip

parsley	scarf	quart	horse
varsity	starfish	thwart	indorse
	parfait	shorten	endorse
harsh		important	morsel
marsh	carve	quartz	corsage
partial	starve	mortal	torso
	marvel	tortoise	horseshoe
arch	harvest	assorted	horseback
starch		shorthand	
parch	[ɔr]	shortcake	contortion
march	or	mortify	warship
large	matador	forty	
charge	humidor	quartet	scorch
barge	nor		torch
margin	for		blowtorch
	war	cord	fortune
harp		lord	
sharp	xx	ward	gorge
sharpen		ordeal	George
carpet	New York	ordain	forge
	cork	coordinate	
garb	stork	cordial	warp
barb	fork	accordian	torpedo
carbon	pitchfork		
marble	orchid		absorb
garbage	porcupine	horn	warble
barbecue		corn	orbit
	morgue	acorn	morbid
arm	organ	scorn	
harm	organic	adorn	storm
alarm	organize	born	windstorm
charm	organdy	morn	norm
farm	mortgage	thorn	form
army		warn	deform
armistice	cohort	ornate	uniform
garment	contort	ornament	platform
farmhouse	sort	cornet	conform
pharmacy	short	tornado	inform
	cavort	morning	warm

lukewarm	snore	seaport	source
normal	lore	support	force
formal	folklore	davenport	divorce
informal	galore	sport	foresee
warmth	deplore	passport	foresight
torment	explore	export	foursome
Formica	implore	import	porcelain
formation	floor	fort	
formula	soar	portal	
formulate	sore	portable	porch
deformity	shore	porthole	
conformity	ashore	deportment	
	pore	fourteen	doorman
dwarf	pour	fortnight	foreman
wharf	outpour		foremost
orphan	downpour	hoard	
forfeit	bore	horde	forth
	more	chord	fourth
north	Baltimore	gourd	henceforth
orthodontist	fore	toward	forthcoming
orthopedic	four	sword	
northeast	before	board	
northwest	pinafore	aboard	[ʊr]
	wore	blackboard	
[or]	swore	ford	you're
		afford	cure
oar		boredom	secure
ore	xx		manicure
corps			obscure
core	horehound	torn	mature
encore	storehouse	lorn	pure
score	forehead	shorn	tour
gore		mourn	detour
tore		worn	endure
store	pork	hornet	lure
door	forecast	forenoon	sure
adore			insure
outdoor	court		poor
ignore	port	hoarse	moor
	deport	course	

130

xx	[aʊr]	xx
yourself	our	hourglass
bourbon	hour	ourselves
gourmet	scour	
	sour	
	devour	

Vowel + [r] + Vowel (The vowel following [r] is noted.)

[r i]

bereave	cemetery	arid	curious
dungaree	terrace	carry	during
nectarine	dairy	carriage	jury
serene	daring	garret	jurist
cerise	derrick	tariff	fury
jamboree	canary	lariat	furious
marine	dictionary	hilarious	original
submarine	imaginary	chariot	arithmetic
farina	millinery	Paris	accurate
	stationary	parish	licorice

[r ɪ]

	malaria	marry	gorilla
	necessary	marionette	terrific
irresistible	commissary	marriage	asterisk
herein	sheriff	starry	notary
bacteria	cherry	safari	lottery
material	cherish	orange	battery
lyric	perish	torrid	mystery
syringe	bury	florid	diary
cereal	berry	sorry	moderate
serial	blueberry	porridge	mannerism
series	blackberry	foreign	celery
serious	mulberry	forest	calorie
cheerio	burial	forage	gallery
period	merry	orient	glossary
spirit	merit	oriental	sensory
experience	demerit	orientation	answering
imperial	numerical	oriole	luxury
weary	ferry	gory	century
query	fairy	auditory	aspirin
airy	very	auditorium	deliberate
area	vary	inventory	marimba
aerial	various	pictorial	limerick
January	aviary	storage	
obituary	wary	glory	[r e]
herring	iris	glorious	derail
solitary	Irish	flooring	earache
military	fiery	florist	erase
voluntary	wiry	boric	berate
commentary	wiring	memorial	terrain

132

irate
tirade
narrate
orate
oration
uranium
hooray
duration
array
arrange
hurray
decorate
obliterate
generate
tolerate
charade
saturate
geranium
parade
operate
apparatus
beret
enumerate

[rɛ]

erect
irrelevant
florescent
arrest
correct
cigarette
direct
parental
operetta

[raɪ]

neuritis
awry

arise
arrive
horizon
derive
summarize
memorize
variety
pulverize
authorize

[ræ]

eradicate
whereas
erratic
tarantula
cataract
ceramic
giraffe
meringue
boomerang
morale

[rɑ]

ironic
garage
barrage
mirage

[ro]

Nero
erode
erosion
hero
heroic
zero
heroine
bolero

arrow
narrow
sparrow
barrow
sorrow
borrow
morrow
bureau
neurosis
arose
aroma
corrode
corrosion
macaroni
casserole
parole
chaperon

[ru]

anteroom
buckaroo
macaroon
kangaroo
peruse
maroon

[rʌ]

erupt
corrupt

[rə]

era
irritate
irritant
irritable
coherence
clearance
sirup

pyramid
appearance
miracle
errand
heritage
herald
heresy
harem
inheritance
terrible
terrify
sterile
ceremony
cherub
parent
peril
imperil
experiment
verify
siren
pirate
piracy
virus
carat
carrot
caramel
caravan
mascara
guarantee
clarity
clarinet
clarify
charity
parrot
paradise
parallel
paralyze
parasite

paramount	horrible	porous	mineral
paraffin	corrugate	forum	natural
apparel	coral	Europe	opera
apparent	correspond	curable	liberal
asparagus	torrent	maturity	admiral
barracuda	laurel	purity	humorous
baritone	majority	purify	glamorous
baron	moral	mural	
barrel	authority	durable	
embarrass	warrant	plural	[r aʊ]
marigold	quarrel	insurance	
maritime	oral	accuracy	
maraschino	choral	mackerel	
marathon	chorus	literal	around
aura	glorify	general	surround
origin	floral	generous	arouse
horizontal	deplorable	ignorance	carouse

[ɝ] + Vowel

[ɝɪ]	[ɝo]	[ɝə]
hurry	burrow	currant
curry	furrow	current
scurry	thorough	currency
blurry		occurrence
flurry		
furry		
worry		
erring		
hurricane		
courage		
encourage		
flourish		

Words Which May Be Difficult at the Beginning of Therapy

[r—r]

rear
regard
regret
retire
resort
repair
report
remark
refrain
refresh
reward
reindeer
raindrop
railroad
rare
recreation
restaurant
referee
reference
raspberry
roar
crisscross
cranberry
grapefruit
strawberry
secretary
contrary
astronomer
appropriate
library
laboratory
eardrum
aircraft
airport
hairbrush
carefree
arterial
artery
cardboard

barnyard
margarine
arbitrate
arboretum
barbarian
armory
armchair
farmyard
carfare
arthritis
orchestra
corduroy
ordinary
ornery
cornstarch
courtyard
courtroom
portray
portrait
corporal
furor
career
aristocrat
directory
honorary
literature
territory
cerebral
paragraph

[r—ɝ]

reader
reaper
remember
river
radiator
razor
rector
regular

register
rattler
rather
rafter
rocker
robber
roller
rower
ruler
rooster
rumor
runner
rudder
rubber
creature
crater
cracker
grocer
trigger
treasure
tractor
transistor
prayer
pressure
proper
brother
firecracker
nutcracker
biographer
photographer
stenographer
outrigger
contractor
astronomer
typewriter
hereafter
garter
charter
barter

martyr
ardor
archer
carpenter
arbor
harbor
barber
carburetor
armor
farther
quarter
order
border
forger
dormer
former
corner
porter
torture
exterior
inferior
erasure
irregular
anterior
terrier
barrier
character
mariner
warrior
operator
moreover
surrender
error
terror
horror
juror
caterer
emperor
refrigerator

136

[ɚ – r]

checkerboard
waterproof
kindergarten
forlorn
perspire
gingerbread
perform

[ɚ – ɚ]

particular
forever

[ɚ – ɝ]

perverse
liverwurst

[r – ɝ]

return
reserve
refer
reverse
prefer

[ɝ – r]

anniversary
circumference
mercenary

introvert
larkspur

nursery
vertebrae

[ɝ – ɚ]

furrier
hamburger
murder
furniture
murmur
fervor
further

k

[k]

Construction of the [k] Word Lists

1. There are four categories:
   a. the [k] followed by a vowel including initial [k] and initial and medial [k] blends.
   b. the [k] preceded by a vowel including final [k] and final and medial [k] blends.
   c. the [k] preceded and followed by a vowel.
   d. initial, medial, and final [k] blends [kr, skr, kl, kw, skw, rk, ŋk, lk, sk]

2. Where appropriate, the [k] is combined with other consonants in the order which follows:

   [h, j, r, k, g, ŋ, t, d, n, l, s, z, ʃ, ʒ, tʃ, dʒ, p, b, m, f, v, θ, ð, hw, w].

   The words kick, king, kit, kid, kin, kill, kiss; or hack, yak, rack, tack, knack, lack, sack, shack, and jack illustrate some of these combinations.

   If a slight shift in vowels is desired, words such as kit, kite, cat, cot, coat, cut, curt, and cute are found in the first half of the list because [k] is combined with [t] after [h, j, r, k, g, ŋ].

3. Where appropriate, the [k] is combined with vowels and diphthongs in the order which follows:

   [i, ɪ, e, ɛ, aɪ, æ, ɑ, ɔ, o, ʊ, u, ʌ, ə, ɚ, ɜ, ɝ, aʊ, ɔɪ, ju].

4. When there are two [k] sounds in a word, the second one is underlined.

5. To facilitate the location of a word in a category, initial [k] blends are noted by x and medial [k] words are noted by xx.

Characteristics and Use of the [k] Word Lists

1. Choose words which are appropriate for the age and interests of the client. Many words are listed for high school students and adults but would not be considered for small children. The lists also reflect the relative frequency of each vowel in combination with [k]. For example, there are many more words beginning with [kæ] than [ki].

2. Determine which sound combination is the easiest.
   a. If it is [k] + Vowel, begin on pages 142—147. Choose the vowel which makes the [k] production easiest. This frequently is [ɔ] or [ɑ].
   b. If it is Vowel + [k] begin on pages 148—152. Choose the vowel which makes the [k] production easiest.
   c. If it is the [ŋk] final blend, begin on page 156.

3. It may or may not be desirable to proceed down the [k] + Vowel list through the medial blends. If it is not desirable, skip to the next list.

4. The initial [sk] blend is listed according to the vowel which follows it because the vowel influences the production of the blend. However, [sk] blend words are easily found because they are listed immediately after initial [k] words.

5. For very young children who substitute [t] for [k], it is usually unwise to choose words containing both the [t] and [k] in the early stages of therapy because they tend to cause confusion if the [k] is not stabilized. For example, the words *cat, coat, cut, talk, take,* and *took* should be avoided.

Methods of Correcting the [k] *Sound*

The auditory-visual method of teaching the [k] is preferred and should be attempted first. However, in some cases, the client is unable to say the [k] without additional assistance. The following ideas have been helpful in these instances.

1. Ask the client to open his mouth as wide as he can and say [kʌ]. This suggestion is particularly good for children who substitute [t] for [k] because it is difficult to say [t] with the jaws in this position. A mirror may be used to observe the elevation of the back of the tongue.

2. Ask the client to push his tongue against the lower central incisors and pretend to be a tongue-tied crow as he says *caw* [kɔ]. It may be necessary to hold the tongue blade down with a tongue depressor.

3. Ask the client to say [tʌ]. Say, "Now make that sound with the back

140

of your tongue." This frequently results in $[k \wedge]$, particularly with older children who have a cleft palate.

4. With your thumb and forefinger, press against the sides of the client's throat at the apex of the neck and jaw and release the pressure quickly as you say $[k \wedge]$. Ask the client to say $[k \wedge]$ as you repeat the pressure and release.

5. Place a tongue depressor on the tongue blade and push the tongue back against the soft palate. Withdraw the tongue depressor suddenly. Ask the client to say $[k \wedge]$ as you withdraw the tongue depressor.

6. Ask the client to prolong the $[\eta]$ sound. Tell him to force a puff of air into his mouth before releasing the $[\eta]$. Have him repeat the $[\eta k \wedge]$ until he can feel the point of tongue and soft palate contact. Ask him to think he is going to say $[\eta]$ and put his tongue in the $[\eta]$ position but instead just say the $[k \wedge]$.

7. Rarely it is necessary to ask the client to gargle water to give him the idea of elevating the back of the tongue. Ask him to pretend to gargle without water. A distorted $[k]$ sound will result at first but, with practice, the $[k]$ can be produced.

[k] + Vowel*

[ki]

			x
key	kindling	asking	skate
keyhole	kill	basket	skein
keen	kilowatt	basketful	scale
keynote	kilt	basketball	scathe
keel	kiln	wastebasket	
keep	killjoy	husky	**xx**
	kiss	musket	arcade
x	kitchen	bearskin	archangel
	kibitzer	sheepskin	fruitcake
ski		napkin	shortcake
skier	**x**	pumpkin	pancake
scheme		bumpkin	encase
skeet	skit		encage
schemed	skid	## [ke]	incapable
	skin		volcano
xx	skill	cake	escape
	skillet	cater	landscape
marquee	skillful	caterer	
mosquito	skip	katydid	## [kɛ]
housekeeper	skim	cane	
	skimp	canine	care
## [kɪ]		kale	caretaker
	xx	case	careless
kick		casing	careful
king	market	chaos	kerosene
kink	orchid	chaotic	keg
kingdom	orchestra	cage	kettle
kingfisher	orchestration	cape	kelp
kit	trinket	caper	ketch
kitten	blanket	capon	kept
kid	junket	capable	chemistry
kidnap	bronchial	cable	kemp
kidskin	onionskin	cablegram	
kin	oilskin	came	**x**
kindergarten	brisket	cambric	scare
kindle	pesky	cave	scary

*Most words ending with s, ed, and ing are not listed but should be considered if additional words are needed.

142

scarce
schedule
skeleton
sketch
skeptic

[kaɪ]

kayak
cayenne
coyote
kite
kind
kindhearted
kaiser
kibosh

x

sky
skies

xx

archive
bronchitis
mankind
womankind
unkind

[kæ]

carry
character
carrot
caravan
cactus
cackle
canker
kangaroo

cat
cataract
caterpillar
category
cattle
caddie
can
canning
cannot
canon
canopy
canister
canyon
can't
cantaloupe
canter
canteen
candy
candid
candle
cancer
cancel
canvas
calla
calico
calorie
calendar
callous
caliber
casserole
cask
casket
cascade
cast
caster
castle
chasm
cache
cash

cashier
cashmere
catch
catcher
casual
cap
capital
captive
capsule
capsize
capture
cab
cabin
cabinet
cabbage
cameo
camera
camp
campaign
campus
campfire
camphor
calf
caffeine
cavern
cavity
calves

x

scat
scatter
scan
scant
scandal
scallion
scalp
scalpel
scab

scabbard
scamp
scamper
scaffold

xx

sarcastic
sarcasm
forecast
outcast
broadcast
wildcat
encamp
volcanic
askance
mascara
foolscap
bobcat
tomcat

[kɑ]

car
caramel
cargo
cart
cartilage
carton
cartoon
cartridge
card
cardiac
cardinal
cardboard
carnival
carpet
carpenter
carbon
carbonate

143

carfare
carve
khaki
cockroach
cocktail
cocksure
cockpit
cog
congress
cot
cottage
cotton
cottontail
cottonmouth
cottonwood
cod
codfish
concave
concrete
contest
contrary
contract
contrast
contradict
concert
concentrate
conflict
conversation
collie
collar
colic
colony
college
column
columbine
costume
cosmetic
cop
copy

copper
cob
cobbler
cobweb
comma
comic
comet
comedy
common
comment
comrade
compound
compact
complicate
combat
combination

x

scar
scarlet
scarf
scarves
scholar
scallop
scald
Scotch

xx

narcotic
sidecar
handcar
handcart
incomplete
melancholy
discard
butterscotch
hopscotch
abscond

caw
corridor
correspond
cork
cord
corduroy
corn
corner
cornet
cornstarch
corse
corsage
cordial
caucus
caught
cauterize
caudle
call
calling
cauliflower
cost
cause
caution
cough
coffee

x

scorn
scorch

xx

incorporate
escort
discord

[ko]

core
corps

court
courthouse
courtyard
courtroom
courtly
coral
chorus
correspond
coarse
course
coerce
coke
cocaine
cocoa
cocoanut
coax
coagulate
coat
cote
code
coed
cone
coincidence
coal
coalition
colon
colt
cold
coast
cosy
coach
coeducation
cooperate
cobalt
cobra
comb
coma
cove

144

x

score	coop	custom	oncoming
scholastic	couth	customer	discolor
scold		customary	discoloration
scone	x	cuspid	discuss
scope		cousin	discomfort
	schooner	cup	discover
xx	school	couple	
	schoolyard	couplet	[kə]
encore	schoolroom	cupful	
bronco	school-teacher	cub	career
bunco	schoolmate	cubbyhole	correct
incoherent	scoop	cupboard	correction
raincoat		come	corral
alcove	xx	cumquat	congratulate
discourse		cumbersome	congratulation
fiasco	air-cool	compass	catastrophe
horoscope		comfort	cadet
periscope	[kʌ]	cuff	canoe
telescope		cover	canary
microscope	cut	covering	canal
fresco	cutting	coverage	continue
fourscore	cutout		content
beachcomber	cutoff	x	contend
topcoat	cutworm		contempt
	cud	skunk	control
[kʊ]	cuddle	skull	contribute
	cunning	sculptor	conduct
cook	country	scum	condition
cuckoo	cull	scuff	condense
could	color	scuffle	condemn
couldn't	color-blind		conceit
cushion	colorful	xx	consider
	cult		conceal
[ku]	cultivate	haircut	consist
	culture	bedcover	conceive
coo	culprit	handcuff	consent
cougar	culminate	income	concern
cool	cuss	incoming	consume
coolie	custard	encumber	
	custody		

145

congeal
confirm
confetti
confide
confine
confess
confession
confuse
convince
convention
collide
cologne
colossal
collision
collusion
caprice
capricious
caboose
commit
committee
comedian
kimono
command
commence
camelia
commission
compare
comparison
compete
companion
compel
compile
compose
comply
complete
complain
complexion
combine
combust

146

cafe
cavort

xx

Arkansas
harken
darken
parka
vodka
tinker
anchorage
inconsiderate
incomplete
welcome
alcohol
alkali
alkaline
alkalize
talcum
balcony
Balkan
falcon
polka
disconnect
discontinue
discontent
episcopal
hibiscus
misconstrue
Alaska
musketeer

[kɚ]
xx

anchor
handkerchief
tanker
whiskers

[kɝ]

cur
curry
curt
curtain
curtail
courtesy
curtsy
curd
currant
current
currency
colonel
kernel
curlicue
curse
cursive
courage
curb
curfew
curve
curvature

x

scurry
skirt
scourge

xx

encourage
discourage

[kaʊ]

cow
cower
cowhide
cowcatcher
count

county
counter
counteract
counterfeit
council
counsel
counselor
cowlick
cowskin
couch
cowboy
cowbell

x

scow
scour
scout
scowl

xx

encounter
discount
miscount

[kju]

cue
cure
curious
curative
curable
cucumber
cute
cuticle
culinary
Cupid

cupola   cubit
cube   cumulate
cubic   cumulous
cubicle

Vowel + [k] *

[ik]

eke
reek
wreak
Greek
streak
freak
teak
antique
sneak
leak
bleak
oblique
seek
sheik
peak
speak
beak
meek
weak
week
tweak

xx

equal
equalize
sequel
sequence
sequin
sequoia
secret
weakling

[ɪk]

rick
derrick

boric
historic
trick
nitric
metric
brick
fabric
tick
hectic
attic
static
mathematic
patriotic
antic
frantic
gigantic
stick
artistic
optimistic
domestic
drastic
fantastic
mastic
rustic
yardstick
lipstick
chopstick
broomstick
Dick
medic
panic
tunic
lick
frolic
public
flick

sick
seasick
basic
music
pick
topic
toothpick
atomic
economic
graphic
thick
wick

xx

strict
restrict
district
predict
depict
perfect
tickle
nautical
article
particle
radical
sickle
bicycle
pickle
nix
six
mix
fix
prefix
betwixt

hickory
dictate
dictator
dictation
dictaphone
nickname
ticklish
eclipse
prickly
bricklayer
recline
becloud
exceed
pixy
excel
excess
except
exception
excite
excuse
exclaim
exclude
sixteen
sixteenth
extinct
extinguish
extortion
extent
extend
extension
exterior
exterminate
extreme
experience
expect
expend

*Words ending with es and ed are not included and should be considered if final [ks] and [kt] blends are desired.

148

expense	beefsteak	direct	text
expel	headache	detect	pretext
experiment	snake	protect	next
expanse	rattlesnake	elect	
expose	lake	intellect	ecru
expound	flake	dialect	recreation
express	sake	select	secretary
expression	forsake	neglect	technical
diction	namesake	sect	detective
dictionary	shake	dissect	elective
fiction	bake	bisect	selective
ricksha	make	insect	objective
exchange	fake	eject	pectin
picture	wake	reject	spectator
mixture		project	necktie
fixture	**xx**	interject	elector
bequeath	acreage	object	directory
chickweed	sacred	subject	necklace
equip	breakdown	aspect	execute
liquid	breakneck	respect	vexation
bequest	makeshift	prospect	extract
equator	brakeman	suspect	eczema
equation		perfect	exhibition
require	[ɛk]	infect	eccentricity
	reck	heckle	hexagon
[ek]	wreck	freckle	flexible
ache	trek	speckle	exsert
rake	shipwreck	hex	exhale
earache	deck	rex	ecstasy
drake	bedeck	pyrex	textile
mandrake	neck	latex	sexton
brake	fleck	annex	sextet
break	peck	silex	electricity
windbreak	henpeck	triplex	extra
take	speck	duplex	electron
heartache	beck	perplex	dextrose
stake		flex	electrify
steak	**xx**	apex	texture
mistake	erect	vex	direction

149

[æk]

election	hack	tract	practical
section	yak	attract	bacteria
ejection	rack	retract	activate
objection	wrack	detract	cactus
lecture	crack	distract	actor
intellectual	wisecrack	subtract	tractor
expedition	track	exact	benefactor
export	tack	tact	actress
expert	attack	intact	factory
	hardtack	enact	exactly
[aɪk]	stack	transact	acne
	knack	pact	jackknife
	snack	impact	acclimate
hike	lack	fact	blacklist
strike	alack	cackle	backlash
trike	shellac	tackle	backlog
tike	plaque	ax	axis
dike	black	tacks	axiom
like	lampblack	tax	accident
alike	sac	lax	accent
ladylike	sack	relax	accelerate
dislike	ransack	wax	access
homelike	shack	beeswax	accept
pike	jack	axle	taxi
bike	lumberjack		taxable
mike	applejack	packhorse	relaxation
Mike	flapjack	blackhead	saxophone
	pack	backhand	packsack
xx	back	acrid	vaccinate
	bareback	acrobat	maximum
motorcycle	fullback	sacrifice	backstage
	horseback	jackrabbit	backstroke
microbe	halfback	blackcap	jackstraw
microfilm	whack	backgammon	backslide
microphone		background	action
likely	**xx**	active	reaction
likelihood		activity	traction
dry-clean	act	practice	attraction
likeness	react		retraction

150

detraction
distraction
fraction
actual
fracture
blackjack
blackball
blackboard
blackberry
backbite
backbone
acme
blackmail
blackfish
sackful
backfire
aqua
aquaplane
aquamarine
backwash
backwater
backwood
backward

[ɑk]

hock
hollyhock
rock
bedrock
frock
shamrock
clock
o'clock
ticktock
stock
dock
knock
lock
deadlock

padlock
bloc
block
hemlock
floc
flock
sock
shock
chock
pock
bock
balk
mock

xx

ox
pox
smallpox
box
tinderbox
hatbox
bandbox
pillbox
mailbox
fox
oxen

blockhouse
octane
octave
October
octagon
octopus
doctor
doctoral
nocturnal
doctrine
chocolate

toxin
toxic
oxide
dioxide
oxygen
approximate
boxer
foxglove
boxwood
boxful
obnoxious
pockmark
lockjaw

[ɔk]

auk
hawk
jayhawk
talk
stalk
beanstalk
chalk
balk
walk
jaywalk
sidewalk
boardwalk

xx

auction
auctioneer
awkward

[ok]

oak
yoke
stroke
broke

soke
soak
choke
joke
poke
spoke
smoke
folk
invoke
woke
awoke

xx

local
focal
bifocal
vocal
hoax

okra
endocrine
localize
vocalize
proclaim
chokecherry

[ʊk]

hook
buttonhook
rook
brook
cook
took
overtook
nook
look
overlook

outlook
shook
book
handbook
passbook

xx

bookrack
bookbinder
bookmark
bookworm

[u k]

duke
fluke
spook

xx

nuclear
nucleus
lukewarm

[ʌ k]

truck
struck
tuck
stuck
duck
luck
potluck
pluck
suck
shuck

chuck
puck
buck
muck
amuck

xx

instruct
obstruct
duct
product
deduct
abduct
knuckle
pinochle
honeysuckle
chuckle
buckle
barracks
lux
flux

destructive
destructible
buckteeth
duckling
huckleberry
knucklebone
huckster
buckskin
destruction
obstruction

deduction
suction
luxury
buckshot
structure
buckboard
buckwheat

[ə k]

haddock
lilac
epoch
stomach

xx

oracle
miracle
obstacle
pinnacle
borax

hypocrite
accredit
autocrat
aristocrat
across
accrue
acknowledge
occlude
acclaim
succeed
galaxy

success
succession
acquaint
antiquate
aquarium
acquire
aquatic

[ɜ k]

irk
dirk
berserk
shirk
jerk
work
network
woodwork
handwork
guesswork
homework
murk

xx

turquoise
semicircle
Berkeley
workhouse
worktable
workday
workshop
workbench
workman

Vowel + [k] + Vowel (The vowel following [k] is noted.)

[ki]

bookkeeper

[kɪ]

ticket
manikin
chicken
picket
despicable
wicket
wicked
trachea
breakage
taking
baking
Viking
racket
racquet
bracket
brackish
lackey
placket
jacket
packet
hockey
rocket
stocking
docket
socket
jockey
pocket
mockingbird
talking
parochial
hooky
rookie
lucky
bucket
akin
anarchist

monarchy
turkey
jerkin
murky
working

[ke]

hurricane
lubricate
lubrication
fabricate
decay
eradicate
medicate
medication
implicate
applique
implicate
became
authenticate
vacate
vacation
decade
stockade
blockade
brocade
locate
location
dislocate
pillowcase
bouquet
bookcase
acacia
occasion
occasional
barricade
masticate
domesticate
vindicate

abdicate
allocate
duplicate
duplication
application
educate
education
educator
stomachache
justification
edification
amplification
altercation
percale

[kɛ]

teakettle
weekend
briquet
biochemistry

[kaɪ]

psychiatry
hawkeye
buckeye

[kæ]

decalcify
decanter
decapitate
handicap
musicale
locality
academy
mechanic
vocabulary

[kɑ]

peacock
economize
apricot
helicopter
pecan
becalm
bicarbonate
go-cart
accommodate
accommodation
accomplice
accomplish
terra cotta
protocol
boycott

[kɔ]

recall
precaution
because
take off
jackal
accord
accordion
accost
holocaust

[ko]

seacoast
honeycomb
echo
psychosis
tobacco
glucose
stucco
Dakota

153

[ku]

recuperate
recuperation
tycoon
raccoon
acoustic

[kʌ]

teacup
hiccup
recover
pickup
become
bicuspid
hookup
accompany
difficult
difficulty

[kə]

deacon
beacon
weaken
ricochet
stricken
predicament
nicotine
licorice
silica
basilica

pelican
sicken
amicable
thicken
breakable
bacon
vacant
waken
awaken
recommend
second
secondary
secondly
impeccable
beckon
mechanism
likeable
acolyte
blacken
jack-o'-
      lantern
macaroni
macaroon
a capella
broccoli
moccasin
hocus-pocus
broken
brokerage
token
locus
locomotive
focus
succotash

buckaroo
buccaneer
America
delicate
applicant
abacus
percolate
mazurka
ukulele
eucalyptus
mucous

[kɚ]

beaker
dicker
snicker
flicker
bicker
acre
acorn
jawbreaker
baker
homemaker
dressmaker
peacemaker
pacemaker
record
woodpecker
cracker
firecracker
nutcracker
lacquer
hijacker

soccer
broker
mediocre
poker
tucker
sucker
seersucker
chucker
pucker
massacre

[kɝ]

recur
occur

[kaʊ]

lookout
account
accountable

[kju]

ridicule
secure
persecute
persecution
peculiar
epicure
barbecue
Dracula
vacuum
evacuate
procure
accuse

[kr]

crease	scream	clay	quench
cream	script	claim	question
Christmas	scribble	clever	choir
crib	scrimp	climb	quiet
crayon	scrape	climate	quite
crane	scraper	class	quack
credit	scribe	clash	quantity
crept	scratch	clap	quality
cry	scrap	clock	quarrel
crime	scramble	clot	quarter
crash	scrawny	claw	quote
craft	scrawl	clause	
crop	scroll	cloth	xx
craw	screw	close	
crawl	scrub	clover	tranquil
cross		clue	banquet
crow	xx	club	headquarters
crocus		cloud	inquire
chrome	discreet	clown	silkworm
crew	ice cream		milkweed
cruel	prescription	xx	
crust	description		[skw]
crutch	manuscript	foreclose	
crumb	postscript	inkling	squeak
crown	discriminate	anklet	squeeze
crouch	discredit	first-class	squint
	discretion	broadcloth	square
xx	ascribe	incline	squad
	describe	include	squash
aircraft	transcribe	inclination	squawk
darkroom	muskrat	tablecloth	squirrel
sauerkraut	escrow		squirt
bankrupt		[kw]	
increase	[kl]		xx
incredible		queen	
woodcraft	clean	queer	disqualify
	clear	quit	misquote
[skr]	cling	quake	
	clip	quaint	
screen	cliff		
screech			

155

[rk] *

perk		
arc		
ark		
hark		
stark		
dark		
lark		
shark		
park		
spark		
bark		
debark		
embark		
mark		
earmark		
watermark		
postmark		
trademark		
landmark		
hallmark		
birthmark		
stork		
pork		
fork		
hayfork		
pitchfork		

xx

sparkle

larkspur
marksman

[ŋk]

ink	trunk
rink	plunk
drink	flunk
brink	sunk
shrink	chunk
stink	junk
link	punk
bobolink	spunk
slink	bunk
blink	chipmunk
sink	
zinc	xx
chink	
pink	wrinkle
mink	sprinkle
wink	tinkle
hoodwink	twinkle
think	periwinkle
yank	ankle
rank	rankle
drank	
prank	larynx
franc	jinx
frank	minx
tank	sphinx
lank	Bronx
plank	
blank	anxious
flank	junction
sank	tincture
shrank	puncture
spank	punctuate
bank	frankfurter
thank	
honk	

[lk]

silk
bilk

milk
buttermilk
elk
talc
sulk
bulk

xx

milkman
bulkhead

[sk]

risk
brisk
frisk
asterisk
disk
obelisk
bisque
whisk
desk
ask
task
flask
bask
mask
husk
brusk
tusk
dusk

*Words ending with ed and s have not been listed but these endings may be added to many of the words above if [kt, ks] blends are needed.

156

[g]

Construction of the [g] *Word Lists*

1. There are four categories:
   a. the [g] followed by a vowel including initial [g] and medial [g] blends.
   b. the [g] preceded by a vowel including final [g] and final and medial [g] blends.
   c. the [g] preceded and followed by a vowel.
   d. initial and medial [g] blends[gr, gl, gw].

2. Where appropriate, the [g] is combined with other consonants in the order which follows:
   [h, j, r, k, g, ŋ, t, d, n, l, s, z, ʃ, ʒ, tʃ, dʒ, p, b, m, f, v, θ, ð, hw, w].
   The words gag, gang, gad, gas, gash, gap, gab, gaff, or hag, rag, tag, nag, lag, sag, shag, bag, and wag illustrate some of these combinations. If a slight shift in vowels is desired, words such as gate, get, got, goat, and gout are found in the first half of the list because [g] is combined with [t] after [h, j, r, k, g, ŋ].

3. Where appropriate, the [g] is combined with vowels and diphthongs in the order which follows:
   [i, ɪ, e, ɛ, aɪ, æ, ɑ, ɔ, o, ʊ, u, ʌ, ə, ɚ, ɜ, ɝ, aʊ, ɔɪ, ju].

4. When there are two [g] sounds in a word, the second one is underlined.

5. To facilitate the location of a word in a category, medial [g] words are noted by xx.

Characteristics and Use of the [g] *Word Lists*

1. Choose words which are appropriate for the age and interests of the client. Many words are listed for high school students and adults but would not be considered for small children. The lists also reflect the relative frequency of each vowel in combination with [g]. For example, there are many more words beginning with [gɑ] than [gi].

157

2. Determine which sound combination is the easiest.
   a. If it is [g] + Vowel, begin on pages 159—160. Choose the vowel which makes the [g] production easiest. This frequently is [ɑ] or [ɔ]
   b. If it is Vowel + [g] begin on pages 161—163. Choose the vowel which makes the [g] production easiest.
   c. If it is an initial [g] blend, begin with that blend on page 166.

3. It may or may not be desirable to proceed down the [g] + Vowel lists through the medial blends. If it is not desirable, skip to the next list.

4. For small children who substitute [d] for [g], it is usually not advisable to choose words containing both the [d] and [g] in the early stages of therapy because they tend to cause confusion if the [g] is not stabilized. Examples of such words are *god, good, dig, dog,* and *dug.*

Methods of Correcting the [g] *Sound*

The [g] is the voiced cognate of [k] Therefore, the suggestions for the correction of the [k] sound made on pages 140—141 would apply to the [g] However, if the client can say the [k], you only need to indicate the addition of voice. If difficulty is encountered, ask the client to put his hand on your throat as you say [gʌ] and then to feel the vibration in his own throat as he says [gʌ].

158

[g] + Vowel*

[gi]

geese

[gɪ]

gear
giggle
guitar
giddy
gill
gilt
guilt
guilty
guild
gizzard
gimmick
gift
give
given

xx

target
bargain
mortgage
headgear
misgivings

[ge]

gay
gait
gate
gaiety
gain
gale
gala

gaze
gage
gauge
gape
game
gave

xx

elongate
elongation
prolongation
engage
nightingale
nosegay

[gɛ]

Gary
garish
get
guess
guest

[gaɪ]

guy
guide
guidance
geyser

xx

disguise

[gæ]

guarantee
gag
gang
gangster
gad
gander
gallery
gallon
gas
gasoline
gasket
gasp
gash
gadget
gap
gab
gaff
gavel
gather

xx

organic
woolgather

[gɑ]

gargle
garter
guard
garden
gardener
gardenia
garnet
garnish
garlic

garland
garbage
garble
garment
got
gotten
god
godsend
godchild
godmother
godfather
gondola
golf
gossip
gosling
gospel
gob
gobble
goblet
goblin

xx

hobgoblin

[gɔ]

gorge
gong
gone
gallstone
gauze

xx

foregone
Bangor

*Most words ending with s, ed, and ing are not listed.

Bengal
disgorge

[goʊ]

go
going
gore
goat
goad
goal
gold
golden
goldenrod
goldfish
goldfinch
ghost
gauche

xx

cargo
embargo
forego
foregoing
outgoing
bingo
tango
mango
congo

[gʊ]

good
goodness

goods
good-bye

[gu]

goose
gooseberry
goof

xx

mongoose

[gʌ]

gutter
gun
gunboat
gunfire
gull
gully
gullet
gulch
gulp
gulf
gust
gusto
gush
guppy
gum
gumdrop
gumbo
guffaw
govern
governor
government

xx

engulf
disgust

[gə]

gorilla
garage
galore
galoshes
gazette

xx

jargon
organ
organize
organdy
disorganize
sorghum
ingot
kangaroo
dungaree
bungalow
fungus

[gɚ]
xx

linger
finger

fingernail
fingerprint
butterfinger
Edgar
hunger
anger
vulgar

[gɝ]

gurgle
Gertrude
gird
girl
gurgitate
girth

xx

schoolgirl

[gɔɪ]

goiter

[gaʊ]

gout
gown
gouge

160

Vowel + [g] *

[ig]

intrigue	prodigal	exalt	integrity
league	jiggle	exhaust	eggnog
colleague	wiggle	exert	exit
		exertion	exile
xx	pigheaded	pigment	eggshell
	bighead	enigmatic	eggplant
eagle	bighorn	enigma	
legal	degree	bigwig	**[aig]**
illegal	regret		**xx**
beagle	degrade	**[eg]**	
	begrudge		tigress
egress	designate	plague	digress
Negro	designation	vague	digression
eaglet	ignite		eyeglass
legalize	ignorant	**xx**	spyglass
	dignity		
[ig]	dignify	fragrant	**[æg]**
	wiggly	fragrance	
rig	neglect	flagrant	hag
prig	igloo		rag
sprig	wiggler	**[ɛg]**	crag
brig	jigsaw		drag
whirligig	exist	egg	brag
dig	exhibit	yegg	tag
renege	exempt	keg	stag
jig	exact	leg	nag
pig	exactly	peg	snag
big	exasperate	beg	lag
wig	exasperation	nutmeg	flag
twig	exaggerate		sag
	exaggeration	**xx**	zigzag
xx	exam	dregs	shag
	examine	segregate	bag
signal	exonerate	segregation	moneybag
wriggle		allegro	

*Most words ending with s and ed are not listed but should be considered for [gz, gd] blends.

161

carpetbag
wag
wigwag
swag

xx

haggle
straggle
bedraggle
waggle

agriculture
aggregate
aggravate
ragtime
dragnet
magnet
magnetic
magnolia
magnify
straggly
flagstone
flagship
bagpipe
magpie
fragment
flagmen
bagman
quagmire
bagful
ragweed
jaguar

[ɑg]

hog
frog

cog
clog
flog
jog
bog
fog
polliwog

xx

boondoggle
joggle

foghorn
progress
bibliography
biography
cognate
incognito
prognostic
prognosis
cognizance
hogshead
cogwheel
hogwash

[ɔg]

dog
bulldog
log
prologue
dialogue
analogue
waterlog

xx

dogcart
dog-tired

augment
dogma
dogmatic
dogwood

[og]

rogue
brogue

xx

program
au gratin

[ʌg]

hug
rug
drug
shrug
tug
dug
snug
lug
slug
plug
chug
jug
pug
bug
firebug
bedbug
doodlebug
humbug
smug
thug

xx

struggle

snuggle
juggle

pugnacious
pug-nosed
ugly

[ɔg]

xx

Portugal

agree
agreeable
aggrieve
disagree
pedigree
filigree
chagrin
integrate
integration
disintegration
emigrate
centigrade
aggression
centigram
diagram
anagram
monogram
milligram
paragraph
autograph
autographic
dictograph
emigrant
aground
diagnostic
diagnose
diagnosis

			[jug]
aglow	undergrowth	burg	fugue
suggest	underground		
[ɚg]		xx	xx
xx	[ɝg]		
wintergreen	berg	burglar	bugle
		burglarize	

163

Vowel + [g] + Vowel   (The vowel following [g] is noted.)

[gi]

yogi

[gɪ]

frigate
digging
piggy
begin
four-legged
bowlegged
agate
ragged
jagged
shaggy
baggage
soggy
dog-ear
dogged
dogie
rugged
nugget
luggage
buggy
forgive

[ge]

regain
brigade
renegade
legation
agaze
agape
corrugate
corrugation
instigate
instigation
castigate
castigation

investigate
investigation
alligator
allegation
delegation
obligation
conjugate
conjugation
forgave

[gɛ]

beget
again
against
together
spaghetti
forget
forgetful

[gaɪ]

beguile

[gæ]

regatta
legality
begat
began
aghast
propaganda

[gɑ]

regard
disregard
cigar
begot
agog
hexagon

pentagon
demigod
forgot

[gɔ]

begone
woebegone
bygone

[go]

ego
seagoing
negotiate
begonia
lumbago
ago
category
pagoda
marigold
ergo
burgomaster

[gu]

lagoon
dragoon

[gʌ]

begun
august
blowgun

[gə]

egotist
egotistic

brigadier
ligament
cigarette
bigot
bigamist
merry-go-round
Copenhagen
pagan
negative
legacy
megaphone
agony
agonize
antagonize
saga
dragon
wagon
diagonal
vagabond
derogatory
derogative
toboggan
August
yoga
bogus
nougat
bugaboo
arrogance
elegance
esophagus
burgundy

[gɚ]

eagre
eager
leaguer

rigor	chigger	dagger	sugar
trigger	vigor	swagger	cougar
outrigger	leghorn	blackguard	braggart
digger	beggar	auger	[gaʊ]
vinegar	tiger	logger	dugout

Initial and Medial [g] Blends

[gr]

greet	angry	glade	triangle
green	hungry	glaze	tangle
grease	congress	glacier	entangle
grin	mongrel	glare	dangle
grill	congruous	glen	jangle
grip	outgrow	glide	spangle
gray	bridegroom	glad	bangle
grade	ingredient	gladiola	mangle
gravy	ingrate	gland	jungle
grind	ingrain	glance	bungle
gripe	engrave	glass	
grime	downgrade	globule	English
grand	congressional	gloss	England
grass	congratulate	glow	angleworm
grab	congratulations	glory	conglomeration
grotto	ingrown	gloat	wineglass
grovel	engross	globe	sunglasses
grow	congruity	glue	
groan	pilgrim	gloom	[gw]
grocer	disgrace	glutton	
grew	disgraceful	glum	guano
group		glove	Guam
groove	[gl]		guava
grunt		xx	
grudge	glee		xx
grumble	glean	tingle	extinguish
ground	gleam	dingle	distinguish
grouse	glitter	single	anguish
grouch	glint	jingle	languid
	glisten	mingle	languish
xx	glib	angle	language
	glimmer	wrangle	bilingual
foreground	glimpse	strangle	penguin

f

[f]

[f]

Construction of the [f] Word Lists

1. There are four categories:
   a. the [f] followed by a vowel including initial [f] and medial [f] blends.
   b. the [f] preceded by a vowel including final [f] and final and medial [f] blends.
   c. the [f] preceded and followed by a vowel.
   d. initial, medial, and final [f] blends [fl,lf,fr, rf,mf].

2. Where appropriate, the [f] is combined with other consonants in the order which follows:
   [h, j, r, k, g, ŋ, t, d, n, l, s, z, ʃ, ʒ, tʃ, dʒ, p, b, m, f, v, θ, ð, hw,w].
   The words fear, fig, fit, fin, fill, fizz, fish, fib; or reef, leaf, sheaf, beef, and thief illustrate some of these combinations. If a slight shift in vowels is desired, words such as leaf, life, laugh, and loaf are easily found because the [f] is combined with [l] after [t, d, n] in each list.

3. Where appropriate, the [f] is combined with vowels and diphthongs in the order which follows:
   [i, ɪ, e, ɛ, aɪ, æ, ɑ, ɔ, o, ʊ, u, ʌ, ə, ɚ, ɝ, ʒ, aʊ, ɔɪ,ju].

4. To facilitate the location of words in a category, medial [f] words are noted by xx.

Characteristics and Use of the [f] Word Lists

1. Choose words which are appropriate for the age and interests of the client. Many words are listed for high school students and adults but they would not be considered for small children. The lists also reflect the relative frequency of each vowel in combination with [f]. For example, there are many more words beginning with [fɪ] than [fu].

2. Determine which sound combination is the easiest.
   a. If it is [f] + Vowel, begin on pages 169—172. Choose the vowel which makes the [f] production easiest.

b. If it is Vowel + $[f]$, begin on pages 173–174. Choose the vowel which makes the $[f]$ production easiest.

c. If it is a blend, begin with that blend on pages 177–178.

3. It may or may not be desirable to proceed down the $[f]$ + Vowel lists through the medial blends. If it is not desirable, skip to the next list.

Methods of Correcting the $[f]$ Sound

The auditory-visual method of teaching the $[f]$ is preferred and should be attempted first. However, in some cases, the client is unable to say the $[f]$ without additional assistance. The following placement ideas have been helpful in these instances.

1. Say to the client, "Bite your lower lip lightly and blow." These instructions may cause an exaggerated movement which is usually adjusted when the words are put in sentences. Use a mirror to observe teeth and lip contact.

2. If the client substitutes $[p/f]$ and retains the substitution in $[f]$ + Vowel words (*fpun* instead of *fun*), Vowel + $[f]$ words will probably be easier. It may be necessary to prolong the vowel before adding the $[f]$. If the $[p]$ substitution persists, place your forefinger on the client's upper lip and inhibit movement. Later the client may inhibit movement of the upper lip with his forefinger until he is capable of voluntary inhibition.

[f] + Vowel*

[fi]

fee	fit	outfit	phase
feat	fitting	codfish	facial
feet	fiddle	goldfinch	fable
feed	fiddler	goldfish	fame
fiance	fiddlestick	inferior	favor
fiend	fin	nonfiction	favorite
feel	finish	infinitive	favorable
feline	fill	configuration	faith
field	filter	confiscate	
feast	filbert	confiscation	xx
feasible	film	elfish	
feature	filth	bullfinch	parfait
feeble	fiesta		barefaced
female	fiasco		about-face
fever	fist	sphere	boldface
	fizz	sphinx	bold-faced
xx	physique		bold-facedly
	fizzle	stratosphere	paleface
airfield	fish	atmosphere	sulphate
outfield	fishy	disfigure	bisulphate
blaspheme	fisher	misfit	disfavor
	fidget	closefisted	
## [fɪ]	fib	blasphemous	## [fɛ]
	fifty		
fear	fifteen	## [fe]	fare
fierce	fifteenth		fair
fearful	fifth	fake	ferry
fickle		fete	farewell
fix		fatal	fed
fiction	xx	fatality	federate
fig		fade	federal
figure	starfish	feign	federation
figurine	blackfish	faint	fend
figment	nonfiction	fail	fence
finger	whitefish	face	fell
fingernail	catfish	facing	fellow
fingerprint			felon

*Most words ending with s, ed, and ing are not listed.

169

felt
fester
festive
festival
pheasant
fetch
feminine
feather
feathery
featherstitch
featherweight

xx

car fare
warfare
heartfelt
bedfellow

[faɪ]

fire
fiery
firearms
firecracker
fireside
fireproof
fireplace
firebrick
fireman
firefly
fight
fidelity
fine
final
find
file
filing

fiber
five

xx

cockfight
gunfire
bonfire
confide
confine
bullfight
satisfy
campfire

[fæ]

faculty
fact
factor
factory
factual
fang
fat
fatten
fad
fan
fantasy
fantastic
phantom
fancy
fanciful
fallacy
facet
fasten
fascinate
fast
fashion
fashionable
fabric

famine
family
famish

xx

unfasten
confab
alfalfa
satisfaction
emphatic

[fɑ]

far
farce
farm
farmer
pharmacy
farmhouse
farmyard
farther
fox
fog
phonic
fond
fondant
fondle
folly
follow
fossil
fob
father

[fɔ]

for
foreign
forest

forage
fork
fort
forty
fortune
form
former
formal
formula
forward
fought
faucet
foster
fawn
fall
falcon
fault
faulty
falter
false

xx

platform
windfall
rainfall
inform
informal
conform
conformation
asphalt
misfortune
transform

[fo]

foe
four
forehead
forecast

forego
fort
fourteen
ford
force
foresee
foresight
forceful
foremost
foreman
fourth
folk
focal
focus
photo
phone
foal
fold
phobia
foam
foment

xx

earphone
headphone
enforce
enfold
unfold
billfold
henceforth
thenceforth

[fʊ]

foot
foothill
footrest
footnote

footlights
footstool
footstep
footprint
football
full
fuller
fullback

xx

barefoot
boatful
handful
spoonful
teaspoonful
tablespoonful
houseful
boxful
dishful
cupful
clubfoot
clubfooted
armful
brimful
mouthful

[fu]

food
fool
foolish

[fʌ]

function
fungus

fun
funny
funnel
fund
fundamental
fuss
fussy
fussed
fusses
fuzz
fudge
fumble

[fə]

ferocious
fatigue
photographer
fanatic
finesse
felicity
facility
facilitate
physician
familiar

xx

orphan
careful
thankful
breakfast
artful
wistful
distasteful
infinite
infant
infantry
infancy

conference
confident
confidence
confidential
alphabet
alphabetic
alphabetize
baleful
willful
useful
wishful
watchful
helpful
emphasis
emphasize
circumference

[fɚ]

forget
forgetful
forgot
forgive
forgiving
forgave
forbid
forever

xx

confirmation
sulphur
camphor
comfort
comforter
comfortable
discomfort

[fɝ]

fir
fur

		[f au]	
furry	infer	fount	funeral
fertile	inferno	found	fuel
fertilize	infirm	founder	fuse
fern	confer	foundation	fusion
furnace	confirm	fowl	fuselage
furnish	transfer	foul	fuchsia
furniture		fouled	future
furlough	[f ɔɪ]		fugitive
first		xx	fume
firm	foyer		
ferment	foil	confound	
fervor	foist	dumbfound	xx
fervid	foible		
further		[f ju]	
		few	confute
xx	xx	futile	confuse
		futility	confusion
headfirst	tinfoil	feud	Confucius
		feudal	transfusion

Vowel + [f] *

[if]	xx	[εf]	[æf]
reef	rift	deaf	half
grief	drift	clef	behalf
brief	snowdrift	chef	raff
leaf	thrift		carafe
relief	gift		giraffe
belief	lift	xx	graph
broadleaf	sift		paragraph
sheaf	shift	heft	dictograph
chief	sniffle	deft	telegraph
beef		left	monograph
thief		cleft	calf
	refrigerate	theft	gaff
	refresh		epitaph
xx	refrain		staff
	different	[aɪf]	distaff
chieftain	defray		laugh
chiefly	defraud	strife	chaff
leaflet	defrost	knife	
beefsteak	befriend	jackknife	
	tutti-frutti	penknife	xx
	nifty	life	
[ɪf]	thrifty	wife	raft
	deflate	housewife	craft
if	diphthong		woodcraft
tariff			graft
sheriff		xx	draft
midriff	[ef]		shaft
skiff		Eiffel	raffle
plaintiff	safe	trifle	baffle
stiff	chafe	stifle	
sniff	waif		after
cliff		lifeguard	afternoon
kerchief	xx	lifetime	aftermath
handkerchief		lifelike	afterward
biff	safeguard	lifesaver	rafter
miff	safety	lifeboat	hereafter
whiff	safety pin		

*Most words ending with s and ed are not listed but if [fs] and [ft] blends are desired, these endings may be added to many of the above words.

thereafter
laughter
craftsman
draftsman
affluence
scaffold
calfskin
halfback
halfway

[ɑf]

doff

xx

waffle

sophomore

[ɔf]

off
cough
take off
checkoff
scoff
cutoff
castoff
layoff
blowoff
show-off

xx

oft
croft
loft

aloft
hayloft
soft
awful

offhand
lofty
awfully
offset
offspring
offshore
offshoot

[of]

oaf
loaf

xx

snowflake
blowfly

[uf]

behoof
roof
proof
waterproof
weatherproof
bulletproof
dustproof
rainproof
bombproof

aloof
pouf
spoof
woof

xx

proofread

[ʌf]

huff
rough
gruff
scuff
tough
stuff
enough
snuff
puff
buff
rebuff
muff

xx

tuft
toughen
ruffle
scuffle
shuffle
muffle

roughhouse
buffalo

muffler
roughshod

[əf]

Joseph

xx

afresh
afraid
affront
diaphram
diaphramatic
afflict
affliction
aflame
afloat
aflutter
cauliflower

[ɚf]

xx

butterfly
overflow

[ɝf]

turf
serf
surf

174

Vowel + [f] + Vowel (The vowel following [f] is noted.)

[f i]

defeat
caffeine
afield

[f ɪ]

prefix
leafy
terrific
scientific
deficiency
Pacific
jiffy
befit
aphid
aphis
crayfish
raffia
graphic
biographic
traffic
taffy
daffy
laughing
prophet
profit
profitable
offing
office
crawfish
coffee
coffeehouse
toffee
trophy
biophysics
bluefish
suffix
puffing
muffin

affix
affinity
affiliate
affiliation
officiate
official
officious
efficient
coefficient
paraffin
microfilm
biography
atrophy
catastrophe
artificial
edifice
benefit
beneficiary
beneficial
crucifix
crucifixion
insufficient
butterfinger
interfere
counterfeit
surface
perfect

[f e]

efface
deface
defame
cafe
cellophane

[f ɛ]

defect
defection

defend
defense
defensible
affair
affect
effect
effective
ineffective
affection
effectual
offend
offense
offensive
inoffensive
profess
professor
profession
perfection

[f aɪ]

refine
citify
defy
define
defile
defiance
sapphire
profile
afire
horrify
terrify
clarify
glorify
purify
petrify
ratify
gratify
identify

notify
certify
beautify
mortify
edify
solidify
modify
signify
magnify
bona fide
nullify
amplify
vilify
qualify
suffice
specify
classify
pacify
crucify
diversify
intensify
calcify
emulsify

[f æ]

artifact
de facto
benefactor
manufacture
butterfat

[f ɑ]

chiffon
befog
afar
safari

175

[fɔ]

reform
deform
default
befall
hayfork
snowfall
guffaw
aeriform
chloreform
perform
performance
waterfall

[fo]

threefold
before
bifocal
afford
microphone
hydrophobia
megaphone
dictaphone
radiophone
telephone
saxophone

[fʊ]

crowfoot
afoot
underfoot
tenderfoot

[fu]

buffoon

[fʌ]

refund
defunct
befuddle

[fə]

peripheral
dutiful
pitiful
plentiful
certificate
stiffen
differential
difficult
difficulty
diffidence
coniferous
chiffonier
playful
effigy
referee
deference
deferential
deafen
definition
deficit
defamation
encephalitis
hyphen

syphon
affidavit
affable
cafeteria
daffodil
laughable
esophagus
often
officer
soften
sofa
roughen
suffocate
insufferable
beautiful
bountiful
modification
edification
elephant
colorful
perforate
perforation
euphony

[fɚ]

defer
differ
differed
Clifford
wafer
effort
heifer
zephyr
offer

coffer
suffer
buffer
biographer

[fɝ]

refer
coiffeur
affirm
affirmative

[faʊ]

afoul
profound

[fju]

refuse
refusal
diffuse
diffusion
effusive
refuge
profuse
centrifuge
curfew
perfume

Initial, Medial, and Final [f] Blends*

[fl]

flee	flew	oneself	fracture
flea	flu	myself	frank
fleet	flute	himself	frankfurter
fleece	fluid	shelf	fragile
fling	flung	golf	frog
flicker	flood	gulf	frolic
flit	flush	wolf	fraud
flip	flamingo	werewolf	frost
flake	flirt	Beowulf	froth
flame	flourish		froze
flavor	flour	xx	frugal
flare	flower		fruit
fleck		wolfhound	fruitcake
fled	xx	twelfth	front
flesh			frontier
phlegm	inflict	[fr]	from
fly	conflict		fraternal
flier	inflate	free	fraternity
flight	inflation	freak	frown
flies	inflame	freeze	
flag	inflammable	friction	xx
flat	influence	fringe	
flannel	sunflower	frill	carefree
flash	cornflower	frigid	breadfruit
flashlight	wallflower	freight	infringe
flow	housefly	frail	confront
flock	pamphlet	phrase	belfry
phlox		frame	Alfred
flop		freckle	bullfrog
florid	[lf]	fret	leapfrog
floss		friend	grapefruit
floor	elf	fresh	[rf]
florist	self	fry	
float	ourself	fright	scarf
flown	yourself	fried	wharf
		fraction	dwarf

*Most words ending with s, ed, and ing are not listed for the initial blends. Words ending with s and ed are not listed for the final blends. If triple blends ending with [ft, fs] are desired, these endings should be considered.

177

⌈m f⌋   xx

nymph   triumphal
lymph
triumph

178

[v]

[v]

Construction of the [v] *Word Lists*

1. There are four categories:
    a. the [v] followed by a vowel including initial [v] and medial [v] blends.
    b. the [v] preceded by a vowel including final [v] and final and medial [v] blends.
    c. the [v] preceded and followed by a vowel.
    d. final [v] blends [rv,lv].

2. Where appropriate, the [v] is combined with other consonants in the order which follows:
    [h, j, r, k, g, ŋ, t, d, n, l, s, z, ʃ, ʒ, tʃ, dʒ, p, b, m, f, v, θ, ð, hw,w].
    The words va<u>n</u>e, va<u>l</u>e, va<u>s</u>e; or <u>r</u>ave, <u>c</u>ave, <u>g</u>ave, <u>kn</u>ave, <u>l</u>ave, <u>sh</u>ave, <u>p</u>ave, <u>w</u>ave, and <u>th</u>ey've illust<u>r</u>ate some of these combinations. If a <u>sl</u>ight <u>sh</u>ift in vowels is desired, words such as v<u>e</u>al, va<u>l</u>e, v<u>i</u>le, and v<u>oi</u>le are easily found because [v] is combined with [l] after [t, d, n] in each list.

3. Where appropriate, the [v] is combined with vowels and diphthongs in the order which follows:
    [i, ɪ, e, ɛ, aɪ, æ, ɑ, ɔ, o, ʊ, u, ʌ, ə, ɚ, ɜ, ɝ, aʊ, ɔɪ,ju].

4. When there are two [v] sounds in a word, the second [v] is underlined.

5. To facilitate the location of words in a category, medial [v] words are noted by xx.

Characteristics and Use of the [v] *Word Lists*

1. Choose words which are appropriate for the age and interests of the client. Many words are listed for high school students and adults but they would not be considered for small children. The lists also reflect the relative frequency of each vowel in combination with [v]. For example, there are many more words beginning with [vɛ] than [vɔ].

2. Determine which sound combination is the easiest.
   a. If it is [v] + Vowel, begin on pages 181—183. Choose the vowel which makes the [v] production easiest.
   b. If it is the Vowel + [v], begin on pages 184—185. Choose the vowel which makes the [v] production easiest.

Methods of Correcting the [v] Sound

The [v] is the voiced cognate of the [f] Therefore, the suggestions for the correction of the [f] sound, made on page 168, would apply to the [v]. However, if the client can say the [f], you need only to indicate the addition of voice. If difficulty is encountered, ask the client to put his hand on your throat as you say [v] and then to feel the vibration in his own throat as he says [v].

[v] + Vowel*

[vi]

vehicle
vehement
veto
venous
Venus
veal
visa
viva

xx

convenience

[vɪ]

veer
vicar
victor
victory
victim
vixen
vigor
vineyard
vinegar
vintage
vindicate
vindictive
viola
villain
village
vilify
viscera
vista
visit
visitor
visible
vicious

vision
visual
visualize
vigil
vigilant
vim
vivid

xx

harvest
invigorate
invincible
invisible
envision
envy
envied
enviable
anvil
convict
convince
convivial
elvish
salvage
obvious

[ve]

vacate
vacation
vacant
vague
vagrant
vain
vane
vein
vale

veil
vase
vapor
vaporize

xx

starvation
convey
inveigle
salvation

[vɛ]

vary
very
variant
various
variation
variable
variability
verify
vex
vet
veteran
veterinarian
venue
venerate
venerable
vent
ventilate
ventilation
ventricle
vend
vender
vendetta
venison

venture
vengeance
venom
velvet
vessel
vest
vestige
vegetarian
vegetate
vegetation
vegetable

xx

corvette
advent
adventure
invariable
invent
inventor
invention
inventive
envelop
invest
investigate
invested
investment
convex
convent
convention
conventional
circumvent

[vaɪ]

vie
via

*Most words ending with s, ed, and ing are not listed.

181

virus
Viking
vying
vital
vitamin
viaduct
vine
vial
vile
violet
violate
violin
violinist
violent
vice
vise
vice versa
visor
viper
vibrate
vibration
vibrant
vivacious

xx

advice
advise
adviser
advisable
environ
environment
invite
grapevine

[v æ]

vacuum
vaccinate
vaccination

vagabond
vat
van
vanity
vanish
vantage
vandal
vandalize
valley
value
valuable
valor
valet
valid
validate
valedictorian
valiant
valentine
valance
valve
vast
vacillate
vaseline
vascular
vamp
vampire

xx

advantage
disadvantage
advance
invalid

[v ɑ]

varnish
varsity
varmint
vodka

volley
volatile
volunteer
voluntary
voluble
volume
volcano
volcanic
vomit

xx

involuntary
involve

[v ɔ]

vault

[v o]

vocal
vocalize
vocation
vogue
vote
vaudeville
volt
volition

xx

invoke

[v ʌ]

vulcanize
vulgar
vulgarity
vulnerable
vulture

invulnerable
convulse
convulsion

[v ɔ]

variety
veracity
vocabulary
veneer
vanilla
validity
valise
velocity
velour
vicinity

xx

carven
larva
advocate
advantageous
invitation
inventory
invalid
envelope
convalescence
canvas
galvanize
pulverize

[v ɚ]

Virginia
verbose

xx

advertise
advertising

			[v ɔɪ]
advertisement	versus	adverb	void
Denver	versify	invert	voile
conversation	version	inverse	voice
culvert	virtue	convert	voyage
silver	virtual	convertible	voyager
silver-plate	virtuoso	converse	
silverware	verge	conversion	xx
	virgin	converge	
[v ɝ]	verb	convergence	invoice
vertical	vermin		envoy
vertigo	verve	[v aʊ]	convoy
vertebra			
verdict	xx	vow	[v j u]
verdant	adverse	vowel	
verse	adversary	vouch	view
versatile	adversity	voucher	

Vowel + [v] *

[iv]

eve	imperative	cursive	pave
heave	nutritive	expensive	wave
bereave	executive	offensive	waive
grieve	consecutive	inoffensive	they've
greave	derogative		
retrieve	negative	xx	xx
reprieve	connotative		naval
breve	consultative	drivel	
naive	additive	shrivel	favorite
leave	native	civil	
relieve	alternative		## [εv]
believe	infinitive	privilege	xx
cleave	relative	positively	
sleeve	positive	civilize	devil
deceive	motive	civilization	daredevil
conceive	locomotive	chivalry	bedevil
achieve	formative		level
weave	primitive	## [ev]	bevel
we've	furtive		
	effective	behave	every
xx	destructive	misbehave	everyday
	festive	rave	everybody
evil	captive	crave	everything
medieval	adaptive	grave	everywhere
weevil	live	deprave	everyone
	olive	brave	beverage
evening	outlive	cave	reverence
Cleveland	sieve	concave	chevron
eavesdrop	missive	gave	Chevrolet
	impressive	forgave	revelation
## [ɪv]	decisive	knave	devilish
	passive	nave	devilment
give	elusive	lave	devilfish
forgive	abusive	conclave	
curative	effusive	slave	## [aɪv]
operative		shave	I've
			hive

*Words ending with s and ed are not listed but should be considered if [vz] and [vd] blends are desired.

arrive	calve	sovereign	move
derive	salve	novelty	remove
contrive			
strive	xx	[o v]	[ʌ v]
drive			
deprive	haven't	rove	of
thrive	ravel	grove	dove
archive	gravel	trove	love
dive	travel	drove	glove
endive	gavel	cove	foxglove
nose-dive		dove	shove
connive	average	clove	above
live	maverick	mauve	
alive	javelin	wove	xx
chive	avalanche		
five	travelogue	xx	covering
	traveler		dovecote
xx	cavalry	oval	dovetail
	cavalcade		aboveboard
rival		[u v]	
			[ɜ v]
ivory	[ɑ v]	behoove	
rivalry		you've	curve
lively	suave	groove	conserve
driveway		prove	reserve
	xx	approve	preserve
[æ v]		reprove	deserve
halve	novel	disprove	observe
have		improve	nerve

185

Vowel + [v] + Vowel   (The vowel following [v] is noted.)

[vi]

reveal
ravine
intravenous
Genevieve
intervene

[vɪ]

previous
abbreviate
leaving
cleavage
deviate
devious
weaving
evict
rivet
revision
trivial
giving
thanksgiving
misgiving
living
livid
Bolivia
oblivion
civic
aviary
aviation
gravy
saving
navy
heavy
crevice
levy
chevy
bevy
ivy
private

avid
having
scavenger
lavish
savvy
savage
novice
soviet
jovial
loving
covet
divinity
division
divisible
individual
television
civilian
severe
persevere
pavilion
dervish
service
fervid

[ve]

evade
evasion
prevail
ave
ovation
avail
available
availability
derivation
deprivation
excavate
excavation
cultivate

cultivator
cultivation
captivate
innovate
innovation
renovate
renovation
elevate
elevation
enervate
enervation
surveyor
conservation
survey

[vɛ]

event
eventual
eventuality
revenge
prevent
prevention
develop
development
November
avenge
severity
intervention
effervescent

[vaɪ]

devitalize
revise
revive
device
devise
divisor
bovine

provide
improvise
divide
divine
survive
survival
supervise
supervisor

[və]

Eva
even
diva
Geneva
derivative
charivari
frivolous
given
nativity
captivity
divot
dividend
carnivorous
livable
pivot
ambivalence
equivalent
haven
raven
craven
evident
evidence
Evelyn
evolution
heaven
revenue
revolution
irreverence

prevalence
brevity
devastate
inevitable
eleven
eleventh
several
seven
seventy
seventh
longevity
privacy
driveable
saliva
enliven
avarice
avocation
avenue
havoc
ravenous
gravity
cavity
cavalier
davenport
navigate
lava
lavender
clavicle
avocado
providence
Java
impoverish
cloven
woven
interwoven
souvenir
juvenile
rejuvenate
movable

coverage
governor
lovable
servant
observant

[vɚ]

beaver
fever
river
liverwurst
deliver
sliver
shiver
quiver
flavor
saver
favor
disfavor
waver
quaver
ever
evergreen
everglade
everlasting
whoever
forever
whatever
endeavor
never
nevertheless
nevermore
whenever
lever
clever
sever
whatsoever

whensoever
wherever
driver
diver
avoirdupois
cavern
tavern
over
overalls
overcast
overcoat
overtime
overtake
overdo
overlay
overlook
oversee
overture
overjoyed
overpass
overbearing
overflow
overweight
moreover
layover
allover
clover
passover
popover
Hoover
maneuver
louver
hover
cover
recover
bedcover
discover
govern
government

lover
fervor

[vɝ]

revert
reverse
reversal
reversible
proverb
avert
averse
aversion
introvert
controversy
controversial
divert
diversify
diversion
diverge
anniversary
perverse

[væ]

evangelic
devaluate
devaluation
evacuate
evangel
evangelist
evaluate
evaporate
prevaricate
divan
bivalve
caravan
cravat

[vɑ]	[vo]	[vɔɪ]	[vju]
evol_ve	evoke	devoid	preview
revol_ve	revoke	avoid	review
devol_ve	revolt		interview
bravado	devote	[vaʊ]	
boulevard	devotion	devout	
samovar	bravo	avow	
[vɔ]	provoke	disavow	
au revoir	divorce		
cavort			

Final [v] Blends

[rv]			dissolved
carve	scarves	resolve	absolved
starve	starves	dissolve	elves
	dwarves	absolve	delves
xx	[lv]		ourselves
carved	delve	xx	shelves
starved	shelve	delved	wolves
carves	twelve	resolved	

188